WE950
mat.
(3)

SWNHS

D1628065

A Podiatrist's Guide to Using Research

Library
Know─┤e Spa
H

Library
Knowledge Spa
Royal Cornwall Hospital
Treliske
Truro. TR1 3HD

For Elsevier:

Commissioning Editor: Robert Edwards
Development Editor: Rebecca Gleave
Project Manager: Nancy Arnott
Designer: George Ajayi
Illustrations Manager: Merlyn Harvey
Illustrator: Precision Illustration and David Banks.

KSpa

A Podiatrist's Guide to Using Research

Ian Mathieson PhD BSc (Hons)

Senior Lecturer, Wales Centre for Podiatric Studies, University of Wales Institute, Cardiff, UK

Dominic Upton PhD FBPsS

Head of Psychology and Health Sciences, University of Worcester, Worcester, UK

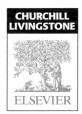

CHURCHILL
LIVINGSTONE

ELSEVIER

EDINBURGH LONDON NEW YORK OXFORD PHILADELPHIA ST LOUIS SYDNEY TORONTO 2008

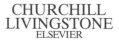

CHURCHILL
LIVINGSTONE
ELSEVIER

An imprint of Elsevier Limited

© 2008, Elsevier Limited. All rights reserved.

No part of this publication may be reproduced, stored in a retrieval system, or transmitted in any form or by any means, electronic, mechanical, photocopying, recording or otherwise, without the prior permission of the Publishers. Permissions may be sought directly from Elsevier's Health Sciences Rights Department, 1600 John F. Kennedy Boulevard, Suite 1800, Philadelphia, PA 19103-2899, USA: phone: (+1) 215 239 3804; fax: (+1) 215 239 3805; or, e-mail: *healthpermissions@elsevier.com*. You may also complete your request on-line via the Elsevier homepage (http://www.elsevier.com), by selecting 'Support and contact' and then 'Copyright and Permission'.

First published 2008

ISBN 10 0-443-10381-X
ISBN 13 978-0-443-10381-0

British Library Cataloguing in Publication Data
A catalogue record for this book is available from the British Library

Library of Congress Cataloging in Publication Data
A catalog record for this book is available from the Library of Congress

Notice
Knowledge and best practice in this field are constantly changing. As new research and experience broaden our knowledge, changes in practice, treatment and drug therapy may become necessary or appropriate. Readers are advised to check the most current information provided (i) on procedures featured or (ii) by the manufacturer of each product to be administered, to verify the recommended dose or formula, the method and duration of administration, and contraindications. It is the responsibility of the practitioner, relying on their own experience and knowledge of the patient, to make diagnoses, to determine dosages and the best treatment for each individual patient, and to take all appropriate safety precautions. To the fullest extent of the law, neither the publisher nor the editors assumes any liability for any injury and/or damage.

The Publisher

ELSEVIER your source for books,
journals and multimedia
in the health sciences

www.elsevierhealth.com

Working together to grow
libraries in developing countries

www.elsevier.com | www.bookaid.org | www.sabre.org

ELSEVIER   BOOK AID
International   Sabre Foundation

The
publisher's
policy is to use
**paper manufactured
from sustainable forests**

Printed in China

Contents

Acknowledgements

This project has been a major undertaking for both of us and has involved the reading and reviewing of a considerable number of research and review papers published in podiatry, medical psychology and physiotherapy journals, texts and websites for both researcher and practitioner. This reading has helped us identify some of the key issues facing podiatrists the country over. We obviously thank the researchers, clinicians and policy makers for all this work and the contributions they have made to the current knowledge base. On a more personal level, several key colleagues have acted as informal reviewers for each of our chapters – they have provided honest and robust reviews of our work for which we are truly thankful (although sometimes we felt the bruises!). They have spotted errors and inconsistencies that were inevitable during the first draft – we hope that we have ironed them all out during this final, published, version. However, if any errors remain we accept, of course, ultimate responsibility.

Many thanks also to Robert Edwards and his team at Elsevier for helping us through this project. Finally, we also thank those in the production of the project – the designers and production editors for enhancing the text with some excellent features, which we hope has provided guidance, direction and added value to all readers.

We must also offer thanks and acknowledgement to those that have provided the support both at work and at home. First, thanks to our friends and colleagues at the University of Wales Institute, Cardiff (UWIC) where both of us were based at the initiation of this project. Subsequently, colleagues (of DU) at the University of Worcester for help, advice, friendship and practical guidance. Obviously, we would also like to thank our many students. Some were excellent students – we learnt from you. Some were terrible and made us think and made us work harder. Some were there begrudgingly but we hope at the end of the sessions you appreciated the value and experience of research and the role it has to your professional practice.

Finally, we would like to thank our families for bringing us sustenance and calming us down during our manic periods when we could think of nothing else other than 'the book'. So special thanks to Nicola, Fraser and Laura and to Penney, Francesca, Roseanna and Gabriel.

Chapter 1

Introduction:
What this book can do for you

The fact that an opinion has been widely held is no evidence whatever that it is not utterly absurd.

Bertrand Arthur William Russell

BACKGROUND TO THIS BOOK

Over the past two decades the importance of research and evidence based practice in podiatry has come to the fore, with the past 5 years seeing it move rapidly up the political agenda. There is now a clear expectation on both the practising clinician and the academic researcher to appreciate the importance of research methods, the value of evidence-based practice and their role in promoting clinical effectiveness. These principles are continually stressed and their role in NHS practice has become ever more developed. Allied health professionals, including podiatrists, have adopted these principles and have recognized their value in developing a high-class, patient-centred service (Upton & Upton 2006).

The need for healthcare research has been widely promoted and this has been reflected in strategy and policy developments in the National Health Service (DH 2000, 2003, NHSE 1998). These policy developments, by their very nature, lead to requirements on all healthcare professionals to develop both a research capacity and an evidence base for effective practice, specifically in our case, for allied health professionals (e.g. The Culyer Report, DH 1994). For example, Rafferty et al (2003) highlighted the requirement to 'upgrade the research capacity in nursing and allied health professions to an internationally acceptable level of quality for all health professions that can meet the needs of the service'. This leads on to the requirements for the allied healthcare professional to undertake and be actively involved in research. As Hicks and Hennessy (1997, p. 597) state: 'If the intention is to move towards an evidence based culture, it is essential that a critical mass of health care professionals is either in a position to conduct research or to implement scientific findings.'

However, there is a need to ensure that we do not view allied health-care professionals as a homogenous research group: for some groups there is a significant body of clinical evidence and research studies (e.g. in physiotherapy, nutrition and dietetics) with groups of active researchers promoting and delivering the evidence base. In contrast, there are pro-fessional groups that have less of a research history and lack a core cadre of researchers and funding (HEFCE 2001). It is likely that podiatry was (and is?) in this latter group until relatively recently. However, this situ-ation is changing and developing, and there is now a strong podiatry presence in successful research centres across the UK. These include the Rheumatology Rehabilitation Research Unit at Leeds University, the Centre for Rehabilitation Sciences at Teesside University, the Centre for Rehabilitation and Human Performance Research at Salford University and the HealthQWest programme in Scotland. The body of podiatric research evidence is growing (Green 2005), and must continue to do so, becoming more specific in order to be valued by both clinicians and aca-demics. Therefore, it is incumbent upon all podiatrists to use the best available evidence and to update and sustain research and practice. This involves, for example, knowledge of National Service Frameworks and Care Pathways, and the underpinning evidence.

Obtaining this research evidence is not simply about conducting research trials and doing ad hoc research – it is about developing the 'reservoir' of knowledge about healthcare. There is a need to bridge the gap between knowledge and practice by strengthening the impact that research has on practice and policy (and, of course, on policy makers; Hanney et al 2000). It is apparent, therefore, that podiatrists need to be both researcher producers and research consumers. In order to be effect-ive at both, a certain level of skill and understanding is required: this book aims to provide this threshold level of understanding. In order to go further and become active researchers, there will also be a need to under-stand the intricacies of research which can be found in a number of other more advanced research texts (e.g. Polgar & Thomas 2000). However, it is the contention that this level of skill is not required for most podiatric clinicians but that a certain knowledge and understanding as a *research consumer* is required.

Furthermore, the development of research is not simply about the reading of journal articles or complex texts, it is about developing links between research and practice by forming relationships between researchers, academics and clinicians in such a way as to develop and provide access to both a clinical and a research infrastructure and atmos-phere. In order to both achieve and improve these links there is a need to attract researchers that can understand the language of evidence and research: this text aims to facilitate this entente cordiale. The movement and discussions between practitioners and academics, or between the applied and theoretical areas of work, has to be encouraged.

There are, of course, some cultural differences between the two groups in terms of the values given to certain skills. For example, the academic may be forced to contribute towards the research assessment exercise (RAE). The RAE requires evidence of publications in peer-reviewed journals which are of a theoretical significance compared to the presentation of research-based evidence for practice which receives little RAE credit for publications elsewhere. However, these forms of presentation and publication may be of more interest and more value to the clinician. We hope to show in this text that this need not be the case and that the practising podiatrist can understand both clinical and basic research in order to fully involve evidence-based practice.

Hence, we are arguing that this distinction may be a false one: research evidence produced in the academic arena can be translated into practice research. The practice-based clinician must value and integrate the academic research. Although this is widely acknowledged, the research suggests (ironically not read by many!) that, in many cases, staff may rely predominantly on experience rather than evidence and that new evidence takes time to enter effective practice. This is no longer a sustainable position for healthcare practitioners, and podiatrists must, and do, accept this development. But additional skills and knowledge need to be facilitated – hence this book.

This text focuses on research skills for healthcare professionals and specifically podiatrists. The central premise of the book is that a majority of healthcare professionals are not active researchers but have to be active research consumers. This is an underlying tenet of modern healthcare that has its roots in the outcomes movement and evidence-based practice. This demands that clinical practices be underpinned by supporting research and consequently even though clinicians are unlikely to be involved in original research, they must be capable of understanding, critiquing and employing information from original research to consolidate and develop their own practice. This book clearly differentiates between the *active researcher* and the more frequent *research consumer*, and aims to increase the confidence with which the 'ordinary' healthcare professional approaches published research. It begins by presenting the five steps of evidence-based practice. Skills in formulating clear, relevant and answerable questions are discussed initially, followed by a 'how to' guide to conducting a literature search. The critical evaluation of the literature identified by a thorough and systematic search is then approached. This step is crucial since the literature base for each profession is rapidly expanding, and it can be difficult to judge which research should be used to inform clinical practice. Making informed decisions about which research contains sufficient validity and reliability (i.e. methodological value) to warrant its use to inform clinical practice is challenging and an understanding of research methods is invaluable for the clinician approaching this task. Whilst there is overlap between the research knowledge required by active researchers and clinicians, traditional texts fail to make this distinction explicit – which means that the needs of the latter group are rarely fully met. The unique aspect of this book is that it acknowledges that research methods need to be placed in the context of the process of evidence-based practice. This means delivering 'bottom line' information, regarding, for example, the weaknesses of a particular study and the consequences of modifying practice despite these weaknesses. This fosters an understanding of the implications of research concepts for the individual clinician, and increases the confidence with which they can approach their professional literature base and use it to inform practice.

IS THIS BOOK FOR YOU?

The book aims to appeal to podiatrists by introducing research in a simple, pragmatic manner that justifies why the topic is vital to you, and provides the information you need in an appropriate way. Whilst books are available on both evidence-based practice and research methods, there are no texts that bridge the two disciplines and discuss research in the *context* of evidence-based practice. Research is a subject often seen by healthcare professionals as peripheral to their core clinical skills, despite the emphasis placed on it in modern healthcare. This book is targeting the majority of podiatrists – clinicians, researchers, academics and students. Hence it is for all those who are involved in clinical practice, not just research, and for those that need a pragmatic guide that acts as a 'how to' manual. Arguably, research has failed to 'make it to the masses', despite this being necessary for evidence-based practice to impact on routine care provision. This text seeks to make research clinically relevant to everyday practice. Hence, to return to the question: 'Is this book for you?', if you are working in podiatry, plan to work in podiatry, are researching in podiatry or are involved in developing podiatry policy, then the answer is yes. The text is for those involved in all aspects of podiatric practice.

This book is different from others: the focus is for the research consumer (which all health professionals must be to help them offer the best treatments to their patients) and in particular the podiatric research consumer. We also hope that this text will be of use for the *active researcher* (a minority of specialists who actively participate in research and operate within a research environment) or those that aspire to be active researchers. The current healthcare provision environment and the demands it places upon health professionals will be discussed as it forms the background scenery for this book. We hope that those clinicians and practitioners who work in this environment will recognize the environment and the tips and advice we offer.

STRUCTURE OF THIS BOOK

We thought long and hard about the structure of this book and it has evolved over its writing to the present state. At the outset, we knew the content, we knew how we wanted to present the material, we knew the order of the material and we thought we knew the structure. So what was our problem? The difficulty was in the individual chapters – how could we differentiate the material, indeed should we differentiate it? We were aware that the research process can be fractioned and this is a particular logic that could provide a final chapter structure. However, we were also aware that the research/evidence-base process should be considered holistically. We had difficulty in differentiating the chapters and in deciding the limits of each chapter – on several occasions we split and then reformed the chapters. Consequently, we hope that you appreciate the chapter structure but also appreciate the 'wholeness' of the research process.

Ultimately, the final chapter structure we settled on, following this first introductory chapter, was as follows.

CHAPTER 2: WHAT IS IT ALL ABOUT?

This chapter introduces the five steps of the process of evidence-based practice (EBP), discussing its relevance in modern healthcare, misconceptions surrounding it and the advantages that it offers. It raises some controversies, but resolves these objectively to demonstrate that employing the approach is useful to the daily work of all podiatrists.

CHAPTER 3: A GOOD ANSWER NEEDS A GOOD QUESTION

This chapter focuses on the first step of the EBP process – formulating questions that will permit a fruitful, appropriately focused literature search to be undertaken. It introduces the *PICO* approach – *Patient*, *Intervention*, *Comparison*, *Outcome* – and provides examples of good and bad questions. This is the essential first step in the whole evidence-based process and this chapter outlines the skills known in yr to get this process right.

CHAPTER 4: THE TRUTH IS OUT THERE

Literature searching is the second step of the process of EBP and requires knowledge of the 'hierarchy of literature' sources to show where to look for information, the ability to formulate search strings to ensure a fruitful search, and knowledge of electronic databases and how they operate. This chapter covers these topics, again drawing specific examples from particular podiatric practical examples.

CHAPTER 5: SEPARATING THE WHEAT FROM THE CHAFF

This chapter begins by presenting evidence that adopting a formal approach to critical appraisal makes it more likely that our analysis of a particular article will mirror the appraisal of experts. It discusses prominent critical appraisal systems that are available and briefly discusses the major issues on which these systems focus. It provides brief information on the points that each system evaluates, but concludes that critical appraisal requires knowledge of research methods. At this point in the text we exemplify the strong relationship between evidence-based practice and research methods before moving on to Chapter 6 which presents a focused discussion of research methods.

CHAPTER 6: THE WHY AND THE WHAT OF RESEARCH

This chapter provides information on research methods from a perspective that focuses specifically on understanding issues relevant to critical appraisal. It considers topics such as research designs and their characteristics, including a discussion of the scope and utility of qualitative and quantitative research designs. Sample selection and the process of randomization, power calculations, measurement reliability and validity, descriptive statistics and inferential statistics are introduced, and the analysis of diagnostic tests considered. All these issues are considered in a brief, focused manner. Case studies are used to show how specific research questions can be tackled, from inception to analysis.

CHAPTER 7: DON'T LOSE IT, USE IT!

The bottom line is that our critical appraisal should provide us with information that will permit us to change our practice. This chapter considers what it would take to convince us to actually change our practice and how we should go about it. It suggests that the evidence required to make us change is context dependent – where lives are at risk then it is a grave, serious decision. However, when we are dealing with relatively minor pathologies where limited efficacious treatments exist, then it is reasonable to change on the basis of weaker evidence. However, the concept of systematic changes that are fully rationalized and monitored are emphasized to take away the subjectivity and randomness that can often occur.

CHAPTER 8: WHAT DIFFERENCE DOES IT MAKE?

If we change our practice then we have a responsibility to monitor the effects of the change, and this leads naturally into outcomes measurement. This chapter focuses on basic issues of audit, how it differs from research and why it is important. It demonstrates that evidence-based practice is a process that is intended to improve our practice and that systematic measurement of outcomes is the only way to achieve this.

CHAPTER 9: DOING IT AT WORK

This chapter explores the difficulty in undertaking and applying research in the NHS. The Research Governance Framework will be outlined and how this can influence research and practice. The importance of such an approach and the impact on the practising professional will be outlined and emphasized. How research can be explored and taken into account when research hits practice is stressed.

CHAPTER 10: WHAT IT WAS ALL ABOUT

This final chapter explores the whole nature of research methods and evidence-based practice: What was it all about, what should I remember, what should I do now? The book then ends with useful resources that can continue the research education process.

FEATURES OF THIS BOOK

Various pedagogic devices have been included in this text with the intent of focusing the reader, reiterating the relevance of key points and acting as a revision device. For example, this includes 'key concept' boxes, 'case studies', 'clinical tips' and 'future research and reading'. Links to contemporary literature will be made and studies drawn from the professions' research base in order to exemplify issues. Importantly, the clinical examples provided come from our practice and have been selected because they present clear examples of how research and evidence-based material can be applied to podiatrists. However, these clinical examples can also be applied to other professions (e.g. physiotherapy) and the underlying values and principles explored will be relevant to all allied health professionals.

REFERENCES

Department of Health 1994 Supporting research and development in the NHS. Report of the R&D Taskforce (The Culyer Report). DH, London

Department of Health 2000 Meeting the challenge: a strategy for the allied health professions. DH, London

Department of Health 2003 The StLaR HR project – phase one consultation report. September–December 2003. DH, London

Green ML 2005 A train-the-trainer model for integrating evidence-based medicine training into podiatric medical education. J Am Podiatr Med Assoc 95:497–504

Hanney S, Packwood T, Buxton M 2000 Evaluating the benefits from health research and development centres. Evaluation 6:137–160

HEFCE 2001 Research in nursing and the allied health professions; Report of Task Group 3 to HEFCE and the Department of Health. Higher Education Funding Council for England, Bristol

Hicks C, Hennessy D 1997 Mixed messages in nursing research: their contribution to the persisting hiatus between evidence and practice. J Adv Nursing 25:595–601

NHSE 1998 Research and development in primary care: National Working Group Report (The Mant Report). NHSE, Leeds

Polgar S, Thomas SA 2000 Introduction to research in the health sciences, 4th edn. Churchill Livingstone, Sydney

Rafferty AM, Traynor M, Thompson DR, Ilott I, White E 2003 Research in nursing, midwifery, and the allied health professions: a quantum leap required for quality research. BMJ 326:833–834

Upton D, Upton P 2006 Knowledge and use of evidence-based practice by allied health and health science professionals. J Allied Health 35(3):127–133

Chapter 2

What is it all about?

There are costs and risks to every programme of action, but they are far less than the long range risks and costs of comfortable inaction.

John F. Kennedy

LEARNING OUTCOMES

By the end of this chapter you will be able to:
- Define the term 'evidence-based practice'
- Explain the overall aims of the process
- Describe the five individual steps of evidence-based practice
- Debate key controversies surrounding the process
- Discuss the advantages to clinical and professional practice of adopting an evidence-based approach.

CASE STUDY

A 32-year-old man has been experiencing pain at the back of his ankle on and off for 5 years. He consults a podiatrist. During the first consultation the physiotherapist finds out that the pain does not seem to be related to an acute injury, is exacerbated by playing football and has stopped him playing on two occasions. Pain is localized to the body of the Achilles tendon, 2 cm above the calcaneus, and several nodules can be palpated. The podiatrist diagnoses Achilles tendinopathy.

This consultation raises various information needs. Although treatment can be initiated based on experience and current practice, many questions can be developed in relation to this clinical scenario.

For example, the accuracy of any diagnostic features or tests used, the best treatment, the number of treatments required and the prognosis are of vital importance.

Where, and how, can the information required to answer these questions be found?

INTRODUCTION

In Chapter 1 we contended that evidence-based practice differs from what is traditionally termed 'research methods' and represents an approach to practice that is vital for all modern healthcare professionals. Whilst research methods focus on the skills that are necessary to conduct a research project – from formulating a hypothesis and selecting a method, to gathering data and performing statistical analyses – evidence-based practice focuses on skills that help clinicians to gather and use information and knowledge that already exists. Any particular patient that we are faced with in the course of a working day can be used to illustrate the difference between the two approaches. The techniques we use in our day-to-day encounters are based on a complex set of information: current clinical guidelines ± departmental protocols ± our personal experience ± our colleagues' input ± various other sources of information. Whilst such an approach is legitimate, it is important in consolidating and developing our practice that we ask questions about what we are doing. Research efforts are ongoing, and the diagnostic tests and therapeutic approaches we use today will become outdated as they are surpassed by newer, better techniques. This is not a modern phenomenon; it is simply a fact of life. For example, Dr Sydney Burwell, a former Dean of Harvard Medical School, stated in the 1950s that: 'My students are dismayed when I say to them, "Half of what you are taught as medical students will in ten years have been shown to be wrong, and the trouble is, none of your teachers knows which half".' (Pickering 1956). Clearly there is a need to consistently re-evaluate our clinical approach to ensure that we are providing the best available treatments to our patients.

It would simply not be practical, however, for clinicians to design from scratch the research required to provide answers to their questions. This would take an enormous amount of time and money, and patients would suffer. This approach would also be wasteful because the answers to our questions are often already available in the existing literature base. And if the answers to our questions are already available then it is unethical to use valuable resources – including money, our time and patients' time – duplicating existing research. It seems logical that, in the first instance, we should look to the existing literature to determine if the information we require already exists.

Whilst it is easy to say 'look at the existing literature for answers to your questions', this is in reality a daunting prospect. This is illustrated by considering that the Medline database has published over 3 million articles in the past 5 years (Medline 2006; www.ncbi.nlm.nih.gov/entrez), whilst the HighWire Press provides free full-text access to over 1 million articles from 919 journals (HighWire 2006; http://highwire.stanford.edu). Clearly what is needed is a 'plan of attack' – an organized approach to this literature that will help us find what we want, when we want it. This is a major focus of evidence-based practice: it is, first and foremost, a system of approaching the existing literature that increases our chances of getting the information we require. As a precursor to the individual chapters of this book which will focus on the *research skills* that define the process of evidence-based practice, we will first consider the approach holistically, refining a definition, considering arguments presented by both the proponents and critics, and, ultimately, justifying our focus on the process of evidence-based practice.

KEY CONCEPT

> Evidence-based practice is first and foremost a system of approaching a vast healthcare literature base to help us find valid answers to our clinical questions so as to increase the quality of patient care.

DEFINING EVIDENCE-BASED PRACTICE

The original definition of evidence-based practice (EBP) was 'the conscientious, explicit and judicious use of current best evidence in making decisions about the care of individual patients' (Sackett et al 1996). Greenhalgh (2000) argued that numerical measures were such an inherent part of the concept that they should be referred to in the definition. As such, she proposed an alternative definition, describing it as 'the enhancement of a clinician's traditional skills in diagnosis, treatment, prevention and related areas through the systematic framing of relevant and answerable questions and the use of mathematical estimates of probability and risk'. Although this definition may be accurate, it is not immediately applicable to the process as it can be practised by allied health professionals. This is because the mathematical estimates referred to are calculated from data gathered from specific types of research – in particular the randomized controlled trial (RCT). However, there are relatively few, good-quality RCTs available that are relevant to the allied health professions (AHPs). Clemence (1998) argues that this is because the RCT design has not been entirely successful in the AHP arena due to the focus on identifying the single most effective treatment for a condition. Allied health professionals commonly provide complex, multi-dimensional treatments that are not well suited to the RCT design. For example, for the Achilles tendinopathy described in the case study there is no single treatment that would be provided – there are various treatments that would be provided simultaneously. Such treatment regimes are complex, and increase the complexity of the RCT.

Straus et al (2005) present a useful alternative definition that avoids the mathematical estimates required by Greenhalgh (2000) (which may make the process more frightening!), suggesting that 'evidence based practice requires the integration of the best research evidence with our clinical expertise and our patients' unique values and circumstances'. However, the original definition conveys the spirit of EBP adequately. Whilst numbers undoubtedly play an important role, it is our contention that clinicians can enter into the process productively, and with a significant impact on their clinical practice, without necessarily progressing to the calculation of numerical measures.

KEY CONCEPT

Evidence-based practice can be defined as 'the conscientious, explicit and judicious use of current best evidence in making decisions about the care of individual patients' (Sackett et al 1996).

Alternative definitions have been suggested which refer to the use of 'mathematical estimates of probability and risk'. However, it is unnecessary to think of EBP in terms of numbers to understand it and practise it.

THE FIVE STEPS OF EVIDENCE-BASED PRACTICE

Evidence-based practice has been consistently described across the key literature as a five-step process (Greenhalgh 2000, Straus et al 2005):

- *Step 1* involves converting our information needs (e.g. relating to diagnosis, treatment, therapy or prognosis) into a focused, answerable question.
- *Step 2* involves efficient literature searching to identify the best information available to answer the question.
- *Step 3* involves critically appraising this information to determine whether it is sufficiently robust (accurate, valid, convincing, appropriate to our practice) to be used to inform our practice.
- *Step 4* requires us to incorporate the results of our critical appraisal into our clinical practice.
- *Step 5* requires us to evaluate the impact a change in practice has made by comparing the outcomes associated with our old treatment with those associated with the new. This tells us if our new approach is truly beneficial or if it is unsuitable for using in our situation.

One of the strengths of this process is its simplicity. For example, a majority of us will have been using libraries for many years and may assume because of this that we already know how to search for and access literature. However, the enormity of the literature base that we must navigate means that specialist skills, exceeding those associated with the use of a traditional library, are required. This point is illustrated by conducting a simple internet search for 'healthcare informatics', which reveals many undergraduate and postgraduate programmes in healthcare informatics offered at various universities. If the content of one of these degree programmes is considered, then we can begin to appreciate just how important it is for us to take literature searching seriously and to devote time to developing skills in these areas. Similarly, we may feel that the way we ask questions about our patients is good enough. However, the process of evidence-based practice teaches us about the vital elements of a question and increases the likelihood of us identifying the precise information we require. Nothing is taken for granted, and we can gain a great deal by learning the specifics of each

CLINICAL TIP

Evidence-based practice is intended to help us provide the most appropriate and most effective treatments for our patients.

step of the process. By devoting a separate chapter to each of these skills, we aim to provide a step-by-step guide which will provide the skills necessary to productively engage in the process.

KEY CONCEPT

To illustrate this process using an everyday example, let us assume that I want to buy a new car. How should I go about deciding which car I should buy? Am I likely to get a car I am happy with if I randomly select five friends or colleagues and ask them what the best car is? How about if I look at the motoring pages of my weekend newspaper? The answer may be yes – I would get a car that I am happy with – but this approach would leave me open to disappointment.

EXERCISE

What are the limitations associated with drawing conclusions from information from a single, subjectively selected, source?

A more considered approach would be to state what I need a car to be, i.e. define what 'best' means when it is applied to me (Step 1).

I would then have to identify the best sources of information to learn about the cars that are available and to refine a short list. This may be magazine reviews, manufacturers' data, independent reviews and owner satisfaction surveys (Step 2).

The data gathered should then be objectively assessed, which would mean evaluating the methods used to draw conclusions and looking for consistency between different sources (Step 3).

I would then have to take the plunge and buy the car (Step 4).

The final step would be to evaluate how well it performed against my needs (Step 5). This would be a continual process, however, and for my next car I can start off from my current car, identify its faults and set out to determine whether there is a better alternative.

THE CHARACTERISTICS OF EBP

For EBP to be successful, some ground rules have to be established. These rules characterize the process of EBP and focus on quality. Quality is a cornerstone of the process, which can be seen to run through all the steps. For example, quality questions must firstly be set to ensure that we are appropriately focused and fully understand our information requirements. Secondly, a good-quality literature search must be planned and conducted to increase our likelihood of identifying the best evidence with which to answer our questions. This is then followed by a critical appraisal of the

CLINICAL TIP

Evidence-based medicine is an aid to clinical practice, not a replacement for a clinician's intuitive ability to get to grips with the idiosyncrasies of daily patient encounters.

research we have found, which again is nothing more than a quality assessment exercise. Since quality is such an intrinsic aspect of EBP there must be some rules about what constitutes good and poor quality and how to integrate quality ratings into the decision-making process.

Research does not simply involve a single approach. There are various methods that we can use to investigate an issue, and our literature search is sure to confirm this by returning everything from case reports to experimental studies for a majority of the search terms we enter. One of the major characteristics of EBP is that it ranks the common research methodologies according to quality. For example, case studies, which are reports that focus on a single patient, are considered a weak form of evidence. This is because we cannot possibly know if our experience with that individual can be used to predict what will happen in the next case or the next 10, 100 or 1000 cases. We have no way of knowing if our case is totally representative or totally idiosyncratic. At the opposite end of the spectrum is the randomized controlled trial (RCT) which is considered a robust research design. These trials, which investigate the effectiveness of treatments, are designed to recruit many subjects and employ a whole range of features aimed at increasing quality. The strict rules of the RCT mean that the results *can* be very useful, because they may be 'generalized', i.e. legitimately applied to other subjects. *Generalizability* (which is technically referred to as *external validity*) is a very important concept which is dependent upon a whole range of factors, and will be discussed more fully in Chapter 6.

The fundamental differences between the common research designs has resulted in them being organized into a pecking order called the 'hierarchy of evidence' (Box 2.1). Case studies sit at the bottom whilst randomized controlled trials sit almost at the top. At the very top we find systematic reviews, which 'do exactly what it says on the tin', by systematically analysing numerous RCTs. A series of questions, derived from a critical appraisal 'tool' such as the CONSORT statement (Moher et al 2001) are then used to quality-rate each study. For example, a study is expected to provide details of the dates that defined the periods of subject recruitment and follow-up to ensure that the study is placed in an appropriate historical context. For each item a score is awarded, and a

---

Box 2.1 The hierarchy of evidence (Greenhalgh 2006)

The hierarchy of evidence is the ranking of research methodologies according to the strength of evidence they are perceived to provide:

- Systematic reviews of multiple randomized controlled trials
- Randomized controlled evidence with definitive results
- Randomized controlled trials with non-definitive results
- Cohort studies
- Case-control studies
- Case series (case studies involving multiple subjects)
- Case studies (involving one patient).

A brief description of each type of study is provided in the glossary, and each design is considered in greater detail in Chapter 6 which deals with research design.

conclusion is drawn on the quality of the evidence provided by each article by considering the total score obtained. If all the trials are rigorous and have come up with the same clear and convincing result, then a strong recommendation can be made. However, when the results of various trials are conflicting, or unclear, it is not possible to make a strong recommendation. Recommendations are an important and intrinsic part of EBP, and represent a holistic appraisal of the available evidence. Appendix 1 provides details of how the levels of evidence associated with individual studies are refined into a 'grade of recommendation'.

CRITICISMS OF EBP

Evidence-based practice is fundamentally concerned with clinical performance and ensuring that we do our best for our patients. If we accept that new techniques are constantly being developed, then we must engage in a process of evaluating new developments to determine whether we should be using them for our patients. Whilst there can be little doubt that a vast majority of clinicians want to do their best for their patients, there is a certain resentment and disapproval of the emphasis that is placed on EBP as a process by which to achieve the best care for our patients. Perhaps the most obvious criticism is that it seems to imply that unless the process is adopted our treatments are inappropriate and based on poor judgement. To understand the true value and application of the process to our practice, it is worth considering not just the advantages, but also the criticisms that have been raised. This should give us a greater, and more objective, understanding of the role of EBP.

An informative discussion of the criticisms of EBP was provided by the CRAP (Clinicians for the Restoration of Autonomous Practice) Writing Group (2002). This article has its tongue firmly in its cheek, but there can be little doubt that it carries a serious message: summarized, that message is that the uncritical, universal, adoption of the principles of EBP undermines professional experience and knowledge, and may be detrimental to patient care. This point was made clearly by Michelson (2003, 2004) in a response to the CRAP Writing Group:

> *During the course of practising orthopaedic surgery (although not documented in the literature), it has been my experience (those of you who adhere to the EBM doctrines will, I hope, excuse this phraseology) that when I hit my finger with a hammer (or mallet, for that matter) my finger hurts. It is even worse if I use a power tool (as in drilling through the finger). My question: how many times do I have to do this before I can say that I have sufficient evidence to potentially causally link the hammer blow to my finger hurting? And what do I use as the control?*
>
> Michelson (2003)

(This comment, which was provided in the form of a rapid response to the CRAP article, clearly struck a chord as he was asked to develop his arguments in an article for the *Journal of Evaluation in Clinical Practice*, which he duly did (see Michelson 2004).)

The Clinicians for the Restoration of Autonomous Practice Writing Group made several points that are worth considering. Firstly, they stated that the 'report' was nailed anonymously to the door of the BMJ for fear of retaliation from the 'grand inquisitors in the new religion of Evidence Based Medicine', indicating that clinicians can feel intimidated by the process of EBP. Secondly, they suggest a list of 10 commandments which may reflect real anxieties that are felt by many clinicians. A few of these are presented in Box 2.2.

Box 2.2 Selected commandments of EBP (CRAP Writing Group 2002)

- Thou shalt honour thy computerised evidence based decision support software, humbly entering the information that it requires and faithfully adhering to its commands.
- Thou shalt neither publish nor read any case reports, and punish those who blaspheme by uttering personal experiences.
- Thou shalt defrock any clinician found treating a patient without reference to all research published more than 45 minutes before a consultation.
- Thou shalt reward with a bounty any medical student who denounces specialists who use expressions such as 'in my experience'.

This literature makes it clear that there are many who are not convinced by the process of EBP. However, it is perhaps harsh to say that they are not convinced and more realistic to state that they are concerned at the sphere of influence that has developed around it. This perspective is supported by Godlee (1998). She acknowledged that the process of EBP was originally intended to empower the common doctor (healthcare professional) by permitting him, with the right training, to understand the evidence supporting a treatment. However, she also conceded that the core principles seem to have developed into a dogma where it now seems that without a Cochrane Collaboration systematic review a treatment is not considered evidence based (Godlee 1998). Such an attitude questions the way that clinicians practise and is quite simply an inappropriate conclusion to draw. As Miettinen (1998) stated: 'Absence of evidence is not evidence of absence [of an effect].'

More critical and academic discussions of the potential dangers of EBP have been provided by various authors (Black 1998, Miettinen 1998, Tanenbaum 1999). They agree that the universal adoption of the process undermines practitioners' personal experience as well as the very nature of professional knowledge. This is because it seems to demand that we practise according to some sort of algorithm which tell us how to act. If this is the case, and all we need to treat patients is the ability to formulate questions, conduct literature reviews and critically appraise the articles found to determine what to do in clinic, healthcare professionals will not be required for much longer. The CRAP Writing Group shares these concerns, predicting that the expansion of EBP will result in the NHS being renamed the National Evidence Service, with 80% of employees' time devoted to generating, analysing and critically appraising evidence, and a cap being placed on the IQ of medical (healthcare?) students!

Although systematic reviews top the hierarchy of evidence, they are a form of secondary research in that they do not conduct the individual research studies themselves, rather they simply review existing research. The major primary research design is the RCT, and although the 'hierarchy of evidence' ranks seven types of study, the reality seems to be that the value and importance of the RCT is overstated whilst other forms of research are underestimated. Black (1998) argued convincingly that this amounts to an appraisal of quality on the basis of the research design, not by how good the study actually was. He went on to demand that 'the quality of evidence should be evaluated not by the method by which it was obtained but by its strengths and weaknesses', and stated that information about clinical decision making was derived from many sources, such as the medical and social sciences, through laboratory research and by skills in diagnosis, among others. This is the approach promoted by epidemiologists, which finds substantial support (Gordis 2000, Vetter & Matthews 1999, Wald 1997). This criticism is recognized by the proponents of EBP, with Greenhalgh (1996) acknowledging that alternative research designs are available which warrant consideration and inclusion in the EBP model, and accepting that systematic reviews must begin to incorporate alternative evidence. It is anticipated that they will begin to incorporate other forms of evidence, but exactly when this happens in a formalized, widespread manner remains to be seen.

CASE STUDY REVISITED

Clinical practice brings a constant stream of information requirements in relation to a majority of clinical encounters. We have two options when faced with these information needs: we can simply continue to practise in the manner we always have, modifying what we do when it seems appropriate. The alternative is to adopt the principles of evidence-based practice, where we utilize a five-step process to think clearly about the information we need in practice, identify this information, appraise it to determine its quality, change our practice where warranted and audit the effects of any changes made. Such a model of practice should be the goal of all clinicians, as it offers the opportunity for enhanced practice.

CONCLUSION

Despite the criticisms of the process of EBP, it seems reasonable to suggest that seeking evidence to support our clinical practice is valuable and can improve the quality of care we provide. Godlee (1998) hit the nail on the head by stating that the core principles of a well-intentioned process have become a damaging dogma. What the balanced, objective clinician needs to do is resolve this controversy by mixing a healthy dose of EBP with a reflective approach to practice which considers the needs of individual patients. The controversies surrounding EBP can be negotiated if we focus on the original intention, approach the process critically and acknowledge that our clinical actions are informed by evidence from various different sources. Knowledge of the dogmas that have developed helps us to get them into perspective and formulate a way forward. EBP is a clearly formulated approach to practice that offers us help and, when viewed as an adjunct to practice as opposed to a modus operandi, has clear clinical application on a daily basis.

REFERENCES

Black D 1998 The limitations of evidence. J R Coll Physicians Lond 32:23–26

Clemence M 1998 Evidence-based physiotherapy: seeking the unattainable? Br J Ther Rehab 5:257–260

CRAP Writing Group 2002 EBM: unmasking the ugly truth. BMJ 325:1496–1498

Godlee F 1998 Getting evidence into practice. BMJ 317:50

Gordis L 2000 Epidemiology. WB Saunders, Philadelphia

Greenhalgh T 1996 Is my practice evidence based? BMJ 313:957–958

Greenhalgh T 2000 How to read a paper: the basics of evidence based medicine, 2nd edn. BMJ Books, London

Greenhalgh T 2006 How to read a paper: the basics of evidence based medicine, 3rd edn. Blackwell Publishing/BMJ Books, Oxford

Michelson J 2003 Evidence based medicine–CRAP should now consider the role of common sense. BMJ 326:602

Michelson J 2004 Critique of (im)pure reason: evidence-based medicine and common sense. J Eval Clin Pract 10:157–161

Miettinen O 1998 Evidence in medicine: invited commentary. Can Med Assoc J 158:215–221

Moher D, Schulz KF, Altman DG 2001 The CONSORT statement: revised recommendations for improving the quality of reports of parallel-group randomized trials. J Am Podiatr Med Assoc 91:437–442

Pickering G 1956 Quote in BMJ:113–116

Pickering G 1956 Cited in Straus S, Richardson WS, Glasziou P, Haynes R 2005 Evidence based medicine: how to practice and teach EBM 3rd edn. Churchill Livingstone, Edinburgh

Sackett DL, Richardson SW, Rosenberg W, Haynes BR (eds) 1996 Evidence based medicine workbook. Churchill Livingstone, Edinburgh

Straus S, Richardson WS, Glasziou P, Haynes R 2005 Evidence-based medicine: how to practice and teach EBM. Churchill Livingstone, Edinburgh

Tanenbaum S 1999 Evidence and expertise: the challenge of the outcomes movement to medical professionalism. Acad Med 74:757–763

Vetter NM, Matthews IP 1999 Epidemiology and public health medicine. Churchill Livingstone, Edinburgh

Wald N 1997 The epidemiological approach. In: Souhami RL, Moxham J (eds) Textbook of medicine, 3rd edn. Churchill Livingstone, Edinburgh

Chapter **3**

A good answer needs a good question

It is not the answer that enlightens, but the question.

Eugene Ionesco

LEARNING OUTCOMES

By the end of this chapter you will be able to:
- Appreciate that formulating a question is the first part of any search strategy
- Clearly formulate an answerable question suitable for searching the literature

- Understand and use the concepts of PICO
- Appreciate the similarity and difference between POEMs, DOEs, COWs, CATs, CAMs and COPEs.

INTRODUCTION

In Chapter 2 we explored the concept of evidence-based practice and the five key steps within this philosophy, and, in particular, how this can be applied within a practice and research setting. When these five steps were outlined and explored it was highlighted that the first step 'involves converting our information needs (e.g. relating to diagnosis, treatment, therapy or prognosis) into a focused, answerable question' (Greenhalgh 2000, Straus et al 2005).

This chapter will explore this first step in more detail and how we can convert our information needs into a clear, focused and answerable question. This involves reviewing the question and refining it until we can search for appropriate literature using a sensible framework. The search for literature must be guided by a question, framing it, and for this search to be efficient and fruitful the question must be appropriately defined. To be blunt, if we want to have a specific answer then we need a specific question.

There are many texts and reports on evidence-based practice and research skills. All emphasize the importance of asking the right question

CLINICAL TIP

We need to ensure that our questions are focused in order to complete an efficient and sensitive search – relate them to your clinical practice for maximum impact.

and most have it emphasized from the outset (e.g. Armstrong 1999, Straus et al 2005). There are some key reasons why it is important that we learn to ask specific questions about practice and why these texts stress this skill so prominently:

- If we want to improve practice it is essential we pose the right questions. If we don't pose sensible questions then we will never get appropriate information in order to make rational change.
- Time can be saved when completing our searches by posing specific questions.
- Learning how to pose questions is essential to the process of lifelong learning and should awaken our 'curiosity and delight in learning' (Richardson 1998).
- Learning how to pose specific questions from our practice is an excellent countermeasure against arrogance, because those who seek answers will discover how tentative our answers are and how much we don't know.
- Learning how to pose a well-built question can foster better communication with other practitioners.
- Vague questions lead to vague answers, specific questions to specific answers.

Case Study

A stocky, well-built, 21-year-old man comes to your service complaining of a painful forefoot after running whilst playing football. He reports a sharp pain in the forefoot that is aggravated by walking and tenderness to pressure on the top surface of the metatarsal bone. On examination you notice diffuse swelling on the skin over the forefoot. Although the man has had an X-ray nothing is apparent but you consider that there is evidence of a stress fracture in the metatarsal bones. Since the patient has some important events coming up he is keen to prevent this from deteriorating. You are worried that this stress fracture may progress to an overt fracture of the bone. You order a bone scan and splint the foot for protection. However, since this man has a previous history of broken metatarsal you decide that a thorough analysis of the running style will be undertaken once the fracture has recovered. You decide to complete two literature reviews on the subject of metatarsal fractures, firstly to explore the link between running and metatarsal stress fractures and, secondly, out of interest to explore whether there is anything (in particular an oxygen tent) that can improve the speed of metatarsal fracture recovery.

FORMULATING THE QUESTION

When completing a literature search there are seven steps that we can see are broadly necessary:

1. Clarify the search question.
2. Identify the most important components for searching.
3. Identify your databases.
4. Translate your concepts into terms used by the database.
5. Identify a range of synonyms to describe your concepts.
6. Combine concepts using Boolean operators.
7. Review the results and revisit steps 1–5 in light of the results.

In this chapter we will explore the first two steps – clarifying the search question and identifying the most important components for searching. Once this has been achieved we will move on to the other elements (i.e. step 3 onwards) in Chapter 4. However, when completing a literature search we must remember our purpose; defining a question for practice may be slightly different from a research literature review and there will be subtle differences in how we frame the question and how we go about addressing it. However, the fundamental points will be the same – the research question is essential!

The key to obtaining a successful search is to understand what you are looking for. In brief, the potential pitfalls to avoid include vagueness, too complicated a research question or more than one question being involved. Using the example of our podiatric chum attempting to find information on stress fractures of the metatarsal, a range of difficulties may be encountered – from too much information to too little. Examples of how extensive this can be can be seen in Table 3.1. If the researcher enters a vague research question, then an unmanageable amount of information is produced. In contrast, if the research question is too narrow, then virtually nothing is returned.

Once you have clarified your question for your topic then you need to break it down into distinct, manageable concepts. Hence, in our example, we have a number of distinct areas that could be investigated in relation to stress fractures of the metatarsal:

- biomechanical analysis
- treatment effectiveness, specifically oxygen tents.

When you set about this search you have to be careful in order to get the right amount of information. You may end up with the right amount of information, or you may get either too much or too little, and it is important you phrase your question appropriately in order to avoid these difficulties. There are techniques that you need to employ to either expand or constrict your search. So, for example, you may wish to restrict the search to certain types of study or certain dates, certain forms of treatment or with different types of patient. All of these can have an impact on

Table 3.1 Amount of information returned from Google Scholar

Question	Problems	Amount of information returned
Treatment for broken toe	Too vague	10 100
Treatment of metatarsal stress fracture in Cardiff School of Podiatry	Too specific	2
Interprofessional team working effectiveness for the treatment of metatarsal stress fractures	Too complex – two questions in one: 'interprofessional working' and 'stress fracture of metatarsal treatment', resulting in nothing!	0

the search strategy, as can the terms we use. Hence, our example above suggested that if we search for 'broken toes' then we get over 10 000 articles from which to select. If we limit this to stress fractures of the metatarsals then we get 1820 and if we refine this further to systematic reviews then we limit our search to a much more manageable 65 items. Alternatively, you could limit it according to the population under investigation. Hence, with our fractures of the metatarsals example, if we limit this to running athletes then we have 628 articles and for fractures of the metatarsals and 'footballers' we have just 207.

You have to decide at this stage how precise you want your literature search to be. A highly sensitive search may identify all relevant studies, but unless it is also specific, a large number of 'false positives' or irrelevant studies will be included as well.

CLINICAL TIP

Think about how you want to either restrict or expand your search strategy.

KEY CONCEPT

There are two related concepts here: *sensitivity* (recall) is the proportion of all relevant studies in the database that your search retrieved; *specificity* (precision) is the proportion of all studies retrieved by your search that are relevant. Table 3.2 illustrates how these concepts are related.

If we look at Table 3.2, we find that if we have a high sensitivity and low specificity then we have an unmanageable number of studies, whereas if we have a high specificity and low sensitivity then we miss many. We should aim for a high sensitivity and high specificity to get the maximum number of relevant studies that are workable. The aim of all literature searching is to optimize both sensitivity and specificity within the limits of a defined research question.

Table 3.2 Relationship between sensitivity and specificity

	No. of relevant studies in database	No. of studies retrieved in search	No. of relevant studies retrieved
High sensitivity/low specificity	100	1500	96
Low sensitivity/high specificity	100	26	24
High sensitivity/high specificity	100	112	91

IMPROVING QUESTION FORMULATION

So how can we prepare an answerable question? You will not be surprised that there are some more initials to help us on our way and these are PICO. PICO stands for Patient/Population/Problem, Intervention or Exposure, Comparison and Outcome (Table 3.3).

Table 3.3 PICO

P	Patient, Population or Problem	What are the characteristics of the patient or population? Population? Age group, gender, socioeconomic group? What is the disease/condition you are interested in? Stage of condition/disease? Healthcare setting: primary, secondary or tertiary care?
I	Intervention or Exposure	Which main intervention, prognostic factor or exposure am I considering (e.g. treat, diagnose, observe)? Drug therapy, surgery, radiotherapy? Level of intervention: frequency, dosage? Stage of intervention: prevention, secondary prevention; advanced? Delivery of intervention: self-medication etc.
C	Comparison	What is the alternative to the intervention (e.g. placebo, different drug, surgery?)
O	Outcome	What are the relevant outcomes (e.g. morbidity, death, complications?) Patient oriented: quality of life, reduction in severity of symptoms, adverse effects? Provider oriented: cost-effectiveness?

Table 3.4 PICO and stress fracture of the metatarsal

P	Patient, Population or Problem	Men with stress fractures of metatarsal
I	Intervention or Exposure	Oxygen tent
C	Comparison	No treatment
O	Outcome	Speed of recovery

There are a couple of other initials you should also consider with PICO and they are WT (*What type of question* are you asking – diagnosis, aetiology, therapy, prognosis, prevention, harm?) and *Type of study* you want to find (what would be the best study design/methodology?). However, PICOWT does not roll off the tongue as well as PICO, so PICO is the acronym that is most often employed. However, sometimes the other elements – what type of question and type of study – can be used to refine the question further. However, more of this later.

Going back to our example, we can apply PICO to our footballer with the stress fracture of the metatarsal (Table 3.4).

EXERCISE

Complete a PICO for our case study, exploring the biomechanical assessment of the patient.

LEARN TO ASK A FOCUSED CLINICAL QUESTION

Clinical questions are framed in terms specific to a particular patient. For example, 'What tests should I order for this 21-year-old footballer with painful fourth metatarsal?' or 'How should I treat this patient with a stress fracture?' or 'How can I improve the running style of this footballer to prevent further stress fractures of the metatarsal?' These questions may be relevant if you are talking to a colleague from either your own or an associated profession. However, when attempting to search the medical literature a search question with more specific detail is required. Currently, as phrased, the question presupposes that you know the patient and their particular circumstances. When attempting to refine this question you need to consider the information source you are using: you are much more likely to get a helpful answer if you ask a more generalizable question. Hence, the question could be rephrased as: 'What is the best test to rule out a metatarsal stress fracture in a young physically active adult?' or 'Does treatment with an oxygen tent speed up recovery from a fractured metatarsal?'

It is in attempting to clarify these questions that PICO comes into its own and each of the individual elements of PICO should be explored in turn. In terms of *population*, this is really a description of the group to which the patient or individual belongs and this may include some of the factors highlighted in Table 3.3: age, gender, ethnicity and stage of disease. The description should be specific enough to be helpful, but not overly specific. You are unlikely to find studies of 'Scouse 21-year-old man' (too specific); describing the population as 'young male' is much more likely to be helpful.

Intervention is, as the name suggests, the description of the test or treatment that you are considering. This may be pharmacological, surgical, behavioural, manual or some other form of intervention. You may also wish to specify the level of intervention, the stage of intervention and how the intervention is to be delivered. For example, in our study we would like to explore the effectiveness (in terms of speed of recovery) of sleeping in an oxygen tent. However, as the patient is a professional athlete then we could also explore effectiveness in terms of cost. *Comparison* is also the alternative to the intervention but not all questions need a comparison. Sometimes clinical questions typically involve two options: is it better to have treatment A or treatment B? It may be that 'treatment B' will be just waiting and seeing. In our example the comparison is the usual treatment which involves splinting and rest.

Finally, the *outcome* should generally be something that matters not only to you, but also to the patient. You may well want to involve the patient in defining the outcome. In Table 3.3 both the patient outcomes (e.g. quality of life, reduction in symptoms, correct diagnosis or the cost) and the provider (or clinician) outcomes (e.g. cost-effectiveness) are highlighted. It is also important that the decision is based on consultation with the patient. For example, the speed of recovery may be more important to some than the cost of the treatment.

As we can see from the individual examples provided, there are a number of different types of question (e.g. effectiveness, prevention, assessment, description and risk). On the basis of these question types and the use of PICO we can develop a grid that can be applied to any clinical problem (Table 3.5).

CLINICAL TIP

Using the PICO approach leads to an efficient and effective search strategy.

Table 3.5 PICO grid

	P	I	C	O
Effectiveness				
Prevention				
Assessment				
Description				
Risk				

EXERCISE

If we look at a couple of examples of these in more detail we can see how PICO can be applied to specific clinical cases in order to improve our question so it becomes more focused for our research strategy.

Case 1

Penelope, a successful podiatrist, presents with a complaint of fatigue and loss of interest in her usual professional and personal activities. She denies any suicidal ideation, and has a normal history and physical examination. After diagnosing her with minor depression, her GP prepares to write a prescription for an antidepressant (a selective serotonin reuptake inhibitor, SSRI). Penelope asks about some form of complementary therapy, in particular St John's wort. The GP is then faced with a particular question: 'Is St John's wort a reasonable choice for this patient?'

- Population: Adults with minor depression
- Intervention: St John's wort
- Comparison: An SSRI
- Outcome: Relief of symptoms

Putting these individual elements together, the question the GP could come up with is: 'Is St John's wort or an SSRI more effective at relieving symptoms in adults with minor depression?'

Case 2

Rosie is a young runner who visits you with a pain that is present when her training run first begins, but then disappears as running continues. There is a tender zone along the medial edge of the tibia and you suggest that it is shin splints. Your initial treatment plan is RICE, but Rosie asks if it is worth her paying for massage and heat treatment.

- Population: Physically active adults
- Intervention: Massage and heat treatment
- Comparison: RICE
- Outcome: Relief of symptoms, speed of relief of symptoms, cost-effectiveness

Putting it all together: 'In patients with shin splints, is massage and heat treatment a more effective treatment than simple RICE?'

Exercise

Case 3

Gabriel George has had back pain for several days now, after a weekend of chopping wood at his house. You wonder whether a muscle relaxant would be helpful.

- Population: ?
- Intervention: ?
- Comparison: ?
- Outcome: ?

Now, put it all together in a single, focused question.

Case 4

Francesca Joans has had persistent heel pain. She wonders if she might have a heel spur and thinks she needs an X-ray. Do you order an X-ray in order to diagnose?

- Population: ?
- Intervention: ?
- Comparison: ?
- Outcome: ?

Now, put it all together in a single, focused question.

CAMs, CATs, COWs, POEMs, COPEs, DOEs AND POEs

When we are formulating a research question using PICO we will ultimately be faced with a range of literature from which to select. Although this will form a major part of Chapter 4 it is worth mentioning it here along with a whole range of initials. As stressed earlier we can expand the PICO to include *type of study*. This may, obviously, be studies that are meta-analyses or randomized controlled trials. However, we can also look at other types of study or reports – those that are appraised summaries of clinically useful information.

POEM (patient-oriented evidence that matters) is an acronym that works best in a health/medical care setting, and for those that do not work in such settings the acronym COPES (client-oriented practical evidence search) may be preferred. This is particularly relevant for those working in social care and is similar to POEMs but can be used by non-medical practitioners. COPES has three essential features: they are posed by practitioners but matter to clients; they have practical importance in several ways; questions can guide an evidence search.

Indeed, there are a number of other acronyms which indicate a pre-appraised summary of clinically useful information although we will not explore these in detail:

- CAMs (critically appraised modules)
- CATs (critically appraised topics)
- COWs (case of the week).

Slawson and Shaughnessy (2000) have reported on an innovative approach to what they call 'information mastery'. Central to this are a series of initials – POEMs, DOEs and POEs. POEM refers to the kind of article that:

- addresses a clinical problem or clinical question that podiatrists will encounter in their practice
- uses patient-oriented outcomes
- has the potential to change our practice if the results are valid and applicable.

DOE stands for disease-oriented evidence. DOEs can often be found in the medical literature, and these forms of 'evidence' can be brought to our attention by commercial medical representatives and entrepreneurs keen for us to change our practice. Obviously, this type of evidence should be taken with a pinch of salt as it is often premature in its conclusion. When POEMs exist, forget the DOEs.

Table 3.6 presents the relationship between POEM/DOE and whether the condition is either common or uncommon. Common conditions are those encountered probably on a fortnightly basis in the typical clinic, while uncommon conditions are those encountered less often.

There is, of course, a third and final kind of article that fills the literature that you may be searching, i.e. POEs (patient-oriented evidence). These are studies which don't have the potential to change our practice although they do have a patient focus. They confirm what we already do and, while important, are not priorities for our reading.

Ethically, morally and professionally you have an obligation to provide the best possible care for your patients and hence to stay up to date with the appropriate research literature and the evidence presented. Obviously, you will also be completing other tasks: patient care, administration, scholarly activity and other such time-consuming activities. These will all impinge on your time and hence since your time is finite (and expensive to you and others) you need to focus your efforts by identifying the POEMs and applying them to common conditions in practice. Indeed, focusing your work on POEMs frees you from reading the majority of the literature, since over 97% of it is DOEs and other material (Slawson & Shaughnessy 2000). This high figure is based on a 6-month survey of some 90 journals. It was found that of the 8047 identified articles there were only 213 POEMs (2.6%). This figure includes both common POEMs (encountered at least once every 2 weeks) and uncommon POEMs (encountered less often than every 2 weeks, but at least once over a 6-month period).

Table 3.6 Relationship between POEM/DOE

	POEM	DOE
Common	Read these!	Dangerous
Uncommon	Read if you have time	Worthless

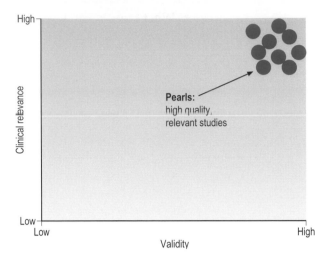

Figure 3.1 Track down the best evidence.

For all of these, particularly DOEs, you should ignore the rare ones – conditions that rarely appear in clinic (or indeed your whole career). However, when you have such a case you should immediately look it up. Common DOEs, since they do not use patient-oriented outcomes, should not change our practice. It is important to remember that much of the medical/podiatric literature is replete with examples of promising data or over-strong conclusions and once further studies were undertaken with patient-oriented outcomes, and more thorough investigations undertaken, then conclusions have been less strong. Have the confidence to reject these findings as premature and stick to tried and trusted evidence. After all, what you are really after are PEARLS (this stands for pearls!) which are high quality, relevant studies (Fig. 3.1). They are studies which have high validity and high clinical relevance. The other types of article are of lesser importance than these.

> **CLINICAL TIP**
>
> Think about what sources you want to review.

YOUR RESEARCH STRATEGY

We have highlighted thus far the formation of an answerable question. This is not, of course, your research strategy complete. This is merely one important step in the formation of a research strategy; indeed, many would argue the most important stage. It is often argued that time spent in this stage will save time later on: better to invest time here than later on dealing with inappropriate data and information.

Your research strategy should consider, alongside the answerable question, answers to the following points:

> **CLINICAL TIP**
>
> Prepare your research strategy in advance.

- Why are you formulating the research question?
- Why do you want to search for information?
- What resources do you have at your disposal?

- What time do you have?
- What are your skills and background – do you want to search podiatry, physiotherapy, medical and nursing literature and so on, or simply limit it to one form?
- How important is the literature review to you?

CONCLUSION

The conclusion to this chapter is relatively straightforward and mirrors that outlined in the introduction: in order to obtain a clear answer you need a clear question. A clear question is essential if we want to save time with our literature search, if we want to improve practice and if we want to enhance our continuing professional development. Overall, it is essential to ourselves, our patients and our service that we have specific answers to our specific questions.

Formulating a question in terms of PICO can be of great help and allows a question to be built using a specific and clearly defined framework. From this the literature and research can flow.

SUMMARY POINTS

- Specific answers require specific questions.
- Your literature and practice search can be negatively affected by a poor question: think in terms of sensitivity and specificity.
- P (Patient, Population, Problem) I (Intervention or Exposure) C (Comparison) O (Outcome) is an acronym that can be used to focus your question.
- Don't forget to consider *what* type of question you are asking and the *type* of study you want to find.
- POEMs and the like can all help in achieving information mastery.

DISCUSSION POINTS

Explore the following cases and develop an appropriate question suitable for completing a research literature review:

1. A 35-year-old man has been experiencing pain at the back of his ankle on and off for 6 years. The physiotherapist diagnoses Achilles tendinopathy and wants to know how best to treat this condition.
2. A 12-year-old girl who goes swimming regularly has been told that in order to prevent development of further verrucae she should avoid swimming baths. She is distraught at this and wants to know the evidence that swimming baths are hosts of the verruca virus.
3. A 42-year-old woman visits you with a fungal nail infection. She has tried oral medication (terbinafine and itraconazole) but these have not been successful. Consequently, ketoconazole is recommended. This has the potential risk of serious liver damage and you are therefore in a quandary: is the risk of the treatment outweighed by the potential benefits?

4. A 14-year-old boy comes to you with athlete's foot. However, he is reluctant to take any medication or apply any 'lotions and potions'. You therefore want to recommend careful cleaning and drying of the feet but are unsure of the evidence.
5. A 43-year-old obese man comes to see you with an excruciatingly painful big toe. You consider it to be a case of gout but want a definitive diagnosis.

REFERENCES

Armstrong E 1999 The well-built clinical question: the key to finding the best evidence efficiently. Wisconsin Med J 98(2):25–28

Greenhalgh T 2000 How to read a paper: the basics of evidence based medicine, 2nd edn. BMJ Books, London

Richardson SW 1998 Ask, and ye shall retrieve. Evid Based Med 3:100–101

Slawson D, Shaughnessy AF 2000 Becoming an information master. J Fam Pract 49(1):1–8

Straus S, Richardson WS, Glasziou P, Haynes R 2005 Evidence-based medicine: how to practice and teach EBM, 3rd edn. Churchill Livingstone, Edinburgh

Chapter 4

The truth is out there

*It is my ambition to say in ten sentences what other men say in whole books –
what other men do not say in whole books.*

Friedrich Wilhelm Nietzsche

LEARNING OUTCOMES

By the end of this chapter you will be able to:
- Identify the key elements of a literature search
- Identify useful sources of information
- Devise and construct a literature search
- Identify appropriate literature from your search that will be relevant to your research question.

INTRODUCTION

CLINICAL TIP

There is a lot of literature out there – we have to think smart and search smart in order to get the appropriate literature.

In Chapter 3 we saw how the research question has to be framed so that you can ask the right question for answering. In this chapter we will explore how the question can be honed down and you can search for appropriate literature. We use the term *appropriate* literature – there is plenty of literature out there (and this chapter will tell you how to find most of it) but not all of it may be relevant. Hence, how can we maximize our literature searches so we get the good stuff and not the irrelevant stuff? However, we also want to ensure that we don't miss that key article or relevant web page that will tell us all we want to know – we have to maximize our inclusivity.

Case Study

A 39-year-old man comes to you with heel pain in his left foot. Background information suggests that this heel pain is of recent onset and has no obvious root in trauma. There is no significant history. He has a rather sedentary job as a university professor and is not involved significantly in any sport. On examination the patient is tall and overweight; there is no indication of any injury or trauma. Your diagnosis is plantar fasciitis which, given your experience, was a relatively simple diagnosis. You suggest exercise and waiting and seeing since, as far as you are aware, there is no other form of treatment for plantar fasciitis. You comment on some forms of treatment to reduce the pain (e.g. ice packs before bed).

However, the professor (being well versed in evidence-based practice!) asks for the evidence for both your diagnosis and treatment plan. You say that this is based on years of experience and having treated plantar fasciitis on a number of occasions. However, your patient questions this and asks you to demonstrate that (a) your knowledge base is up to date and (b) your recommendations are based on best available evidence. You ponder on this for a moment or two, and realize that, indeed, it is some time since you considered the treatment of plantar fasciitis. Consequently, you decide that you want to explore the treatment of plantar fasciitis by undertaking a literature search and devise the following question: 'What is the most effective treatment of plantar fasciitis in a 39-year-old sedentary male?'

SEARCHING THE LITERATURE

You now are ready to commence your literature search (a literature search can be defined as a search for information amongst a range of sources). The first aspect of a literature search is to decide what sources you are going to search and this obviously depends on the reason for undertaking the search. If you are carrying out the literature search for a higher degree or a (hopefully) published article, then it will require a different strategy than if you were preparing for a presentation or attempting to define a new phase of evidence-based practice (as in the case example provided). Sources of literature can encompass both the published and unpublished literature (the latter are sometimes called the grey literature). When we explore the published literature we can also have a variety of different forms of literature – from the World Wide Web to published academic articles. Again, what literature we want to search may be related to the reason that we are undertaking the search. It is apparent that a series of questions must be addressed at the outset in order to best structure your literature search (Brettle & Grant 2004).

WHAT 1?

What is the purpose of the literature search – is it for your practice, for a qualification, for a research project, for a presentation, for a publication? Your answer will provide a framework for the extent of your search.

WHAT 2?

What is your literature search about? What is your research question? As we have seen in Chapter 3, being clear and focused about the topic you are searching through makes it easier to undertake a meaningful search.

WHAT 3?

What are the constraints on your search? Do you have to complete it within the next 5 minutes, 5 hours, 5 days, 5 weeks?

WHAT 4?

What sources are suitable for the topic area? Do you need to search multiple sources? Do you have access to all these resources?

WHAT 5?

What is the extent of your literature search? How comprehensive do you need it to be? Do you need to find one viewpoint? Do you need to find all the literature relating to a particular topic or do you just need to identify the major themes?

When searching for literature you must balance between the sensitivity required and the amount of information available. The more comprehensive your search needs to be, the more sensitive (broad) your search should be. This means that you will need to wade through lots of irrelevant information in order to ensure that you do not miss important data. The aim is to strike a balance between how comprehensive you need to be and what you can manage. However, there are tips for improving the quality of your search so that you get the best available information without out the dross!

CLINICAL TIP

Remember the five Whats!

The responses to these questions will provide you with a guide towards the next stage of the process.

THE RESEARCH QUESTION

In this section the importance of the search *strategy* will be emphasized and it is essential that a strategy is developed rather than lurching from one element to another in a disjointed fashion. There are several steps that can be used in a search strategy and these will be discussed subsequently. However, before beginning your literature search it is important that you have a clear question as was fully discussed in Chapter 3. Completing a literature search is a seven-step process:

1. Clarify the search question.
2. Identify the most important components for searching.
3. Identify your databases.
4. Translate your concepts into terms used by the database.
5. Identify a range of synonyms to describe your concepts.
6. Combine concepts using Boolean operators.
7. Review the results and revisit steps 1–5 in light of the results.

We have already outlined how important the clarity in the search question is along with identifying the important components for searching (see previous chapters), and hence we have already completed the first two steps. We can thus move straight on to step 3 – identifying the right databases.

STEP 3: IDENTIFY DATABASES

Selecting the most appropriate database(s) to search for the job in hand is crucial in literature searching. In podiatry-related research there is a wide variety of databases from which to select. However, databases can offer very different kinds of information. The following are some of the factors to take into account when selecting databases to search.

BIBLIOGRAPHIC OR FULL TEXT DATABASES

Many databases are bibliographic, i.e. they contain citations and abstracts to a variety of articles, for example, journal articles, books, reports or grey literature. The best known example of this type of database in the health sector is Medline, the electronic version of Index Medicus produced by the US National Library of Medicine.

SUBJECT OR METHODOLOGY SPECIFIC AND VALUE ADDED DATABASES

To some extent, all databases are organized along subject lines. Both Embase and Medline are biomedical databases; however, each has strong and weak subject areas within that broad framework. For example, Embase is considered to be stronger in physical and occupational therapy, biology, drug research, psychiatry, health policy and alternative medicine. There are also many databases that focus on a much narrower area of interest such as PsychInfo (psychology).

The main benefit of these databases is that they perform some of the initial sorting of studies, filtering out a specific subsection of the literature that will be of interest to some researchers. The additional benefit is that the compilers may have access to sources outside of the mainstream and may be able to achieve more comprehensive coverage in the topic area than non-specific databases like Medline.

OVERLAP

Overlap is often present between different databases, which can be both positive and negative: positive in that it can help to bring important articles to the widest possible audience; negative in that it can artificially expand the volume of citations to be trawled. It is estimated that overlap between Medline and Embase ranges between 4 and 60%. There are a number of major health-related databases that may be relevant for your search, as follows:

- *Medline*: Bibliographic database produced by the US National Library of Medicine, the electronic version of Index Medicus. Produced from 1966 onwards, it holds citations and abstracts from 4600 journals in 70 countries.
- *Embase*: Bibliographic database produced by Elsevier Science in the Netherlands, the electronic version of Exerpta Medica. Available from 1974 onwards, it contains citations and abstracts from 3800 journals in 70 countries. Its strengths over Medline are its European coverage and inclusion of pharmaceutical topics.
- *CINAHL*: US-produced database of nursing and allied health literature. Coverage is from 1982 onwards and includes citations from

950 journals and publications of the American Nurses' Association and the National League for Nursing.

- *British Nursing Index*: BNI brings together the previously existing Nursing Midwifery Index (NMI), RCN Nurse ROM and Nursing Bibliography. It includes references from 220 health-related journals and has strong UK coverage.
- *AMED*: Allied and Complementary Medicine is a bibliographic database of published journal articles in fields allied to medicine and alternatives to conventional medicine. The database, created by the Health Care Information Service of the British Library, covers a selection of journals in three separate subject areas: professions allied to medicine, complementary medicine and palliative care.
- *Cochrane Library*: The Cochrane Library is an electronic publication designed to supply high-quality evidence to inform people providing and receiving care, and those responsible for research, teaching, funding and administration at all levels. It is available freely in England through the National Library for Health. The Cochrane Library is a collection of seven separate databases: five of these provide coverage of evidence-based medicine; the other two provide information on research methodology. The databases are:
  - Cochrane Database of Systematic Reviews (CDSR)
  - Database of Abstracts of Reviews of Effectiveness (DARE)
  - Cochrane Controlled Trials Register (CCTR)
  - Cochrane Database of Methodology Reviews (CDMR)
  - Cochrane Methodology Register (CMR)
  - Health Technology Assessment Database (HTA)
  - NHS Economic Evaluation Database (NHS EED).
- *PsychInfo*: Bibliographic database of abstracts of articles in the psychological literature from 1800 to date.
- *HMIC*: Three health management databases: Department of Health United Kingdom Library & Information Services, the King's Fund Library & Information Service and the Nuffield Institute for Health.
- *Department of Health Research Findings electronic Register (ReFeR)*: ReFeR is freely available through the National Library for Health. The database provides 'prompt sight' of the findings of completed research from the NHS R&D Programme and the DH Policy Research Programme.

Other specialist databases include:

- *AIDSLINE* – covers AIDS and HIV back to 1980.
- *Allied and Alternative Medicine* – covers complementary and alternative medicine.
- *American Medical Association Journals* – provides the full text of JAMA plus 10 specialty journals produced by the American Medical Association; from 1982.
- *ASSIA* – an applied social sciences database covering psychology, sociology, politics and economics since 1987. All documents have abstracts.
- *Current Research in Britain* – the British national research database of trials in progress.

- *HELMIS* – the Health Management Information Service at the Nuffield Institute of Health, Leeds, UK, indexes articles on health service management.
- *Science Citation Index* – indexes references cited in articles as well as the usual author, title, abstract and citation of articles themselves. Useful for finding follow-up work done on a key article and for tracking down addresses of authors.
- *Toxline* – information on toxicological effects of chemicals and drugs on living systems; from 1981.

EXERCISE

Complete a literature search on plantar fasciitis in sedentary males in a couple of the databases mentioned above: what are the similarities and differences in the literature you obtain?

There is, thus, a considerable amount of information available out there on these databases. However, you can also access further information from other sources. Obviously this will not always be necessary and will be driven by the purpose behind the search. This is not required if you are asking a question about your clinical practice. However, if you are seeking to undertake a complete review (e.g. a systematic review of the literature) then you may want to explore the 'grey literature'. But what is this? While researching your latest paper, project or grant proposal, have you ever spent hours looking in vain for a conference paper or an obscure technical report from a government agency? If you answered 'yes', then you know what it's like to deal with 'grey literature'.

In other words, grey literature is scientific or scholarly literature (e.g. journals and books) published outside normal commercial channels, and could include:

- technical reports from government, business or academia
- conference papers and proceedings
- preprints
- theses and dissertations
- newsletters
- raw data such as census and economic results or ongoing research results.

Searching the grey literature isn't easy. There isn't a 'one-stop shopping' search engine or database that broadly indexes the material the way Medline does for biomedical sciences or CINAHL does for nursing and allied health. Still, if you're hunting for a particular document or you want to see what resources are available on a given topic, there are some places to start. Useful resources for searching the grey literature include:

- *New York Academy of Medicine Gray Literature Report* (www.nyam.org/library/pages/grey_literature_report): A quarterly list of grey literature documents in the field of public health.

- *CRISP Database* (http://crisp.cit.nih.gov): 'CRISP' stands for Computer Retrieval of Information on Scientific Projects. It is a listing of biomedical research projects funded by the US National Institutes of Health.
- *Health Technology Assessment Database* (www.york.ac.uk/inst/crd/htadbase.htm): Large index of reports on healthcare technology trends by government healthcare agencies from around the world.
- *Health Services Research Projects in Progress* (www.cf.nlm.nih.gov/hsr_project/home_proj.cfm): Database from the National Information Center on Health Services Research and Health Care Technology at the US National Library of Medicine.
- *Health Services/Technology Assessment Text* (www.ncbi.nlm.nih.gov/books/bv.fcgi?rid=hstat): Online compilation of various US government reports in the health sciences, focusing on the topics of health services and technology assessment.
- *National Guideline Clearinghouse* (www.guideline.gov): Compilation of clinical practice guidelines from a broad variety of professional organizations and government agencies.
- *National Research Register (UK)* (www.update-software.com/national): Guide to research projects sponsored by, or of interest to, Great Britain's National Health Service.
- *National Library of Medicine's LocatorPlus* (http://locatorplus.gov): Search engine for holdings in the US National Library of Medicine's extensive collection. Good source to look for reports by government agencies. Generally doesn't provide full text access to documents, but an excellent way to see what sorts of government reports exist on a specific topic.
- *World Health Organization current bibliography* (www.who.int/library): Catalogues of publications by the World Health Organization and affiliated agencies, including technical and policy documents.
- *Partners in Information Access for the Public Health Workforce* (http://phpartners.org/guide.html): Nice collection of links to grey literature (as well as some non-grey) resources in public health, including newsletters, reports and guidelines.
- *GrayLIT Network* (www.osti.gov/graylit): Search engine run by the US Department of Energy, intended to provide full text access to government technical reports. Currently participating agencies are the Department of Energy, Department of Defence, Environmental Protection Agency, and the National Aeronautics and Space Administration. Other federal agencies are expected to join as the project expands.
- *Complete Planet* (www.completeplanet.com): A search engine that simultaneously searches more than 70 000 specialized databases and search engines for information on a variety of technical topics. The material contained in these databases and search engines typically does not show up on popular commercial search engines like Google, due to their specialized nature.

As well as identifying the database, it may also be useful to decide what type of literature you want to find – there are many such types of material out there.

EXERCISE

Discuss why the grey literature is important when completing a systematic review.

TYPES OF PAPER IN THE MEDICAL LITERATURE

When you undertake a search of the literature and are reviewing the list of references produced from the database you may find that some (or most?) are not relevant. Consequently, you have to have the skill to review the list of references and identify the references and papers that will be the ones most relevant for you. Sometimes you might be able to do this just by the title, but you should also look at the quality of the paper and the type of methodology. Hence it helps to have some insight into the types of paper that are out there in the literature and how useful they are. The following is a list of the types of article out there, presented in descending order from most to least useful.

REVIEW ARTICLES

These articles can be considered as excellent sources of information and should be viewed as the best place to start your detailed search. These articles are a critical synopsis of the current literature in the particular area of interest and present the professional podiatrist (whether primarily clinician or researcher) with the latest literature. These articles are also useful since they provide an extensive list of useful references that can give direction to your future research. However, a caveat: it is important that you obtain recent review articles since those aged more than a year or two may include old and outdated information rather than up-to-date information with the most recent developments. It must be remembered that for a review article to get into a published journal there can be up to a 12-month time lag. Hence, if the published article is over 2 years old then it is likely to be at least 3+ years out of date. However, a good recent review will contain some worthwhile information on promising developments.

CLINICAL STUDIES

Clinical studies are reports of trials that have been undertaken and which examined the effects of the treatment on patients. For most of those involved in clinical care the decision about the effectiveness of treatment depends on the outcome of prior evidence in human studies. You should try to find papers that are called 'trial' or 'clinical trial' as these include specific useful information.

CASE REPORTS

These articles usually contain reports of an individual case or a limited number of cases of a particular condition or treatment. Because these are reports of *exceptions*, they are not applicable or useful to you unless you happen to be a rare exception as well.

EPIDEMIOLOGY REPORTS

These are reports of the *association* between diverse factors and the incidence of various conditions, illnesses and diseases. Although these reports do not directly prove that factors associated with the condition or illness are actually the cause of the condition, they do provide some indication of the association for future study and investigation.

BASIC SCIENCE

This term covers a range of basic science research – for example, the physiological, biochemical or biomechanical studies that may underlie our practice or a particular podiatric condition. This type of research is extremely important for those attempting to devise new treatments but is of less help to those clinicians trying to find the current best treatment (although it may provide some indication of the 'next best thing').

STEP 4: TRANSLATE YOUR CONCEPTS INTO TERMS USED BY THE DATABASE

We can now move on to the next step and look at how we can translate the concepts into terms used by the database. It should be emphasized that in this chapter we are exploring electronic resource databases, rather than paper based, as these are the predominant forms of database available nowadays.

Once you have identified the concepts for your search you need to translate these into terms that will be recognized by the database. These could be keywords, MeSH (Medical Subject Headings) terms or index terms. This will ensure that you retrieve the articles that are most relevant to your search question. You will need to identify index terms for each of your important concepts.

Some of the databases do all the hard work for you and will suggest the most sensible term you need whereas others allow you to search through the index. On the other hand, others do not provide this feature and you will have to look at how the results have been organised. It is also worth noting that there may be more than one index term that is related to your concept so you may have to select the most appropriate for your search.

To provide an example of this – when exploring the literature you may come across studies that are described as "a double-blind multicentre" or "a double-blind placebo-controlled study" or "a controlled study of". Each of these terms describe what is essentially is a Randomised Controlled Trial (or RCT). So, instead of having to type in each of the phrases in a series of literature searches the indexers of the database will have described this as one single phrase (RCT or Randomised Controlled Trial). This also helps to deal with the subtleties of Anglo-American spelling so Randomised and Randomized are treated the same. Obviously using such terms takes some practice, but it is easy to use and is well worth the effort. There are a series of useful articles that provide all the important information (e.g. Lowe and Barnett, 1994; Greenhalgh, 1997).

STEP 5: IDENTIFY SYNONYMS TO DESCRIBE YOUR CONCEPTS

Although using the **MeSH** (or other index) headings is a useful start it may not always cover your concept in sufficient detail and you may, therefore, have to search using free text. This is also called text word searching and, as the name suggests, involves typing in your term and searching for it in either (usually) the title or the abstract.

There are, of course usually a range of similar words that can be used to describe your concept (i.e. synonyms) underlying your search question. Before you start your literature search you should ensure that these are identified and specified so they can be included within your search strategy. This is important because when you type a free-text word into the database it will usually look for the word exactly as it was typed in. To guarantee that all variations of the words, plurals (e.g. podiatrist, podiatrists) and different spellings (i.e. randomised versus randomized) or concepts (e.g. diabetes, diabetic) are covered then the following features are useful.

TRUNCATION

This feature allows the stem of word to be used, followed by a symbol (usually * or $ – although different databases use different symbols) and identifies all words beginning with that stem to be retrieved. For example diabet* will identify diabetes and diabetic and so on. Care, however, must be ensured to ensure irrelevant articles are not included with too short a stem. For example, rat* would retrieve rat, rats, ratio, rational, rationale, rate, etc.

WILD CARDS

This database feature allows for the replacement of one or (in some cases) more than one letter and search for different spellings. Hence, it might be useful for randomized or randomised by using randomi?ed. Alternatively, wom?n would identify both women and woman.

STEP 6: COMBINE CONCEPTS USING BOOLEAN OPERATORS

You now have a range of ways of describing your search question. To ensure that you retrieve relevant references, you need to combine all these terms. To combine these different concepts in a search you will use Boolean operators. These are logical operators that enable you to broaden or restrict a search. The main operators are 'OR' and 'AND'. These allow you to combine the terms for each of your concepts and then combine them with each other.

A *union* of the sets is created by using the term OR. This new set is created when we combine two or more basic sets using OR. This new set has been created containing all documents in all the selected sets (with the duplicates eliminated). In contrast, when we use the term AND we have the *intersection* of sets. The new set thus created contains only those articles which both sets have in common (again, with the elimination of the duplicates).

USING 'OR'

OR will combine search terms by finding articles that mention *any* of the search terms used. For example, if you search for:

"plantar fasciitis" OR "heel pain"

all the articles that mention plantar fasciitis and all the articles that mention heel pain will be returned, even if the article only includes one of the search terms used (Fig. 4.1).

OR is most useful when you are combining related or alternative terms as part of a sensitive search strategy, otherwise you get too much information.

USING 'AND'

AND combines your search terms by only finding articles that mention *all* of your search terms. For example, searching on:

"plantar fasciitis" AND "treatment"

will only find articles that mention both plantar fasciitis and treatment (Fig. 4.2). It will not find articles that mention plantar fasciitis but not treatment or treatment but not plantar fasciitis. Both terms have to be mentioned in the articles for the article to be included in the results.

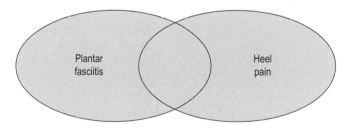

Figure 4.1 "Plantar fasciitis" OR "heel pain".

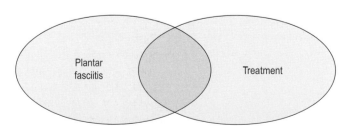

Figure 4.2 "Plantar fasciitis" AND "treatment".

Figure 4.3 'Plantar fasciitis' NOT 'athletes'.

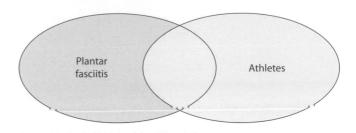

AND is most useful when you are combining different terms in a search and want to limit your search.

USING 'NOT'

NOT isn't available in all search engines, but it is useful to know about it anyway. NOT will eliminate terms from your search. For example, you might want to find an article about plantar fasciitis, but not athletes. A search on:

"plantar fasciitis" NOT "athletes"

will find all the articles that mention plantar fasciitis, but not those that also mention athletes (Fig. 4.3).

NOT is most useful for focussing the results of your search. You would use NOT to eliminate terms you do not want to include in your results.

Note that sometimes speech marks (") have been used – this tells the database to include the term as written. Hence "plantar fasciitis" would find the condition whereas "plantar" and "fasciitis" would get something different.

STEP 7: REVIEWING RESULTS AND REFINING YOUR SEARCH

Once you've combined all your search terms you should have the results you need to answer the question you posed yourself at the start. However, sometimes you might find you have too many or too few results (or even none at all!). When this happens you need to review your search strategy.

If you have too many results you probably need to impose more limits. Think about whether you want to restrict your results to a particular language, type of article, age range or even to a restricted time period (e.g. the last 5 years).

If you have too few results you need to think of other ways to phrase your search or you might need to take out a few search terms. Consider which terms are most important to your search and think of other ways to say them. If, after entering all the terms you can think of, or even searching on just one word, you still have too few or no results, then you have probably found everything that is available through the databases and catalogues.

If, after a search, you get a considerable number of articles that are not relevant to your question, then the term 'NOT' can be used. This term is useful since it allows you to refine your search as you progress. It is much easier to start with a considerable number of articles at the outset and then refine as you go along. It is unlikely that you will produce the perfect article at the outset so you should refine and improve your search as it progresses.

On the other hand, if your search gives you no articles or very few, this may be because of either a flawed search strategy or a flawed indexing system. In order to combat this you may want to adopt a cover-all strategy and search under textwords. For example, the truncation stem 'diabet$' would cover 'diabetes', 'diabetic' and so on, and the term 'podiat$' would cover 'podiatry' and 'podiatric'.

Another useful strategy is to use the 'explode' command as this can help avoid incomplete search strategies. The MeSH terms used are like tributaries from a river: our term diabetes, for example, may be subdivided into 'diabetes in children', 'diabetic foot' and so on. Hence, if you just ask for articles on 'diabetes' you may miss all the articles on 'diabetes in children' unless you explode the term.

SOME OTHER POSSIBLE SEARCHES

Finally, using the concepts described in this chapter, we should simply explore how we can address two simple problems at opposite ends of the extreme. Firstly, you are trying to find a known paper – you vaguely remember when it was produced or who wrote it. By searching the database by field suffix (e.g. *author, title, journal, etc.*) or by *textwords*, the paper can be tracked down. For example, the first step is to get into the database area which covers the approximate year of the paper's publication (you can select either specific years or a range of years). If you are aware of the title of the paper (or a rough approximation) or the journal where it was published, you can use the title and journal search keys or (this is quicker) the .ti and .jn field suffixes. Table 4.1 shows some other useful field suffixes.

Table 4.1 Key concept: Useful search field suffixes (ovid)

Syntax	Meaning	Example
.ab	Word in abstract	fasciitis.ab
.au	Author	mathieson-i.au
.jn	Journal	bmj.jn
.me	Single word, wherever it may appear as a MeSH term	podiatry.me
.ti	Word in title	fasciitis.ti
.tw	Word in title or abstract	fasciitis.tw
.ui	Unique identifier	91574637.ui
.yr	Year of publication	99.yr

In a second case, you really don't know where to start searching. You can use the 'permuted index' option to solve this one – for example, if you wanted to explore the term 'pain' whilst looking to treat our patient with 'heel pain'. This term comes up frequently but searching for particular types of pain would be time-consuming and searching 'pain' as a textword would be imprecise. Hence, we need to understand where in the MeSH index the various types of pain lie, and when we see that, we can choose the sort of pain we want to investigate further. For this, we use the command ptx ('permuted index'):

    1 ptx pain

The screen shows many options, and from this we can select the most appropriate for our needs.

CONCLUSION

This chapter has outlined the importance of developing a literature research strategy, whether for research or clinical purposes. As with many areas of research it is based on solid foundations: the derivation of a sensible and workable research question. Once the question has been derived and clearly specified, you can start on your literature search. Again at this stage you should always keep in mind: Why am I doing this literature search?

The literature search itself is a balance between obtaining all the information you require, but making sure that this does not become extensive and unworkable. The techniques for literature searching have been described and can be implemented with a number of different databases. What is clear, however, is that there is considerable information out there and that the literature search can ensure that you get the maximum benefit from it.

SUMMARY POINTS

- Clearly specify your research question and the reason for undertaking the literature search.
- Remember What, What, What, What and What!
- Any literature search is a balance between sensitivity and specificity.
- There are considerable numbers of databases out there – you have to select the most appropriate one for your needs.
- There are different forms of literature that are published and presented – which you will need to access is dependent on why you are undertaking the literature search.
- The terms in a database need to be clearly specified so that you can translate English into 'database-ese'!
- Wildcards can help with your literature search and Boolean operators can be useful for limiting or expanding the search questions and the consequent extent of the literature found.
- Once you have completed the literature search you should stop and review the material you have found – and re-start if necessary!

DISCUSSION POINTS

1. Why should you prepare a search strategy before you commence a literature search?
2. What forms of literature would you require for a student presentation, a research study and a systematic review?
3. What ways are available to ensure that your literature search is comprehensive?
4. If you obtain excessive material, how can you reduce this to a manageable amount, whilst retaining sensibility and validity?
5. What are the common problems often encountered with literature searching?

REFERENCES

Brettle A, Grant MJ 2004 Finding the evidence for practice. Churchill Livingstone, London

Greenhalgh T 1997 How to read a paper: the Medline database. BMJ 315.180–183

Lowe HJ, Barnett GO 1994 Understanding and using medical subject headings (MeSH) vocabulary to perform literature searches. JAMA 271:1103–1108

Chapter 5

Separating the wheat from the chaff

All truths are easy to understand once they are discovered: the point is to discover them.

Galileo Galilei

LEARNING OUTCOMES

By the end of this chapter you will be able to:
- Discuss what is meant by the term 'critical appraisal'
- Explain the rationale behind the process
- Explain the benefits of adopting a formal critical appraisal tool
- Discuss the range of tools available
- Perform a rudimentary critical appraisal using an appropriate tool.

Case Study

In your daily practice you see many patients with plantar fasciitis, and although you currently utilize a battery of therapeutic measures to tackle the problem, you are aware that there is limited information on the best treatment.

You identify a research paper that you find interesting, which attempts to identify risk factors for this condition. The study describes itself as a 'case-control' design and has been published in a prestigious journal. It claims that reduced ankle joint range of motion, obesity and time spent weightbearing are risk factors for the condition. This seems to suggest that tackling these issues in clinic may be a useful method of treating the condition.

However, you do not quite know what to make of this paper. How should you go about deciding whether the information presented in the paper can be used to inform your clinical approach to plantar fasciitis?

INTRODUCTION

The first two steps of the process of evidence-based practice could be viewed as rather mechanistic. For example, if we learn the key elements that characterize a 'good' question then it becomes relatively straightforward to apply these rules in different situations. Similarly, conducting a rigorous literature review requires knowledge of how to construct a search string and how to use libraries and databases: this knowledge could be regarded as technical, and there are specialists in healthcare informatics who are concerned simply with this skill. These specialists can help us perform a literature search and you may even be fortunate enough to work in an NHS trust which employs specialists in information retrieval to conduct literature searches for staff. This is not to undermine the skills associated with formulating questions and retrieving information; rather it is to suggest that we can fairly quickly develop a working knowledge of these skills.

When we move on to the third step of evidence-based practice we face the altogether more daunting task of having to read and interpret the research we have identified. This process, termed *critical appraisal*, involves a quality assessment of a research study that is aimed at deciding whether it can or should be used to inform practice. This chapter is concerned with the process of critical appraisal and various associated issues; in particular, a series of appraisal 'tools' will be discussed. These are guides which prompt the reader to ask appropriate questions which focus on the major factors determining quality to help us make an informed judgement. However, in the first instance, it is important to consider some issues that will help us get the process in perspective and understand the relevance of the questions set out in the critical appraisal tools.

CRITICAL APPRAISAL: WHAT IT IS AND WHY WE NEED TO DO IT

Critical appraisal is essentially a process of quality and suitability appraisal, whereby we employ a structured approach to evaluating published research to help us draw a conclusion regarding its value to our practice. This is a critical step in the process of evidence-based practice, as it determines whether or not we are going to use the information we have found. However, the need for us to actually conduct a critical appraisal may seem curious: surely if research has been published in a peer-reviewed journal it is a good-quality study with important results? The peer-review process is most definitely helpful in identifying concerns over the quality of published research, but it does not, and cannot, eliminate all concerns that readers may have. This is quite simply because the perfect piece of research does not exist. *All* research involves some element of compromise: researchers operate in a competitive environment where they undoubtedly know what they would like to do, but they also know that due to the constraints placed upon them they will be unable to achieve this, to a greater or lesser extent. For example, funding is rarely ideal – it is likely to be adequate at most – which means that the data collection period may be shorter than desired, there may be fewer subjects involved or their profile may be limited in some way. Whilst the peer-review process goes some way to addressing a range of such issues, they are not familiar with our unique situation – our practice and our patients. It is therefore up to us to critically appraise research to allow us to make an informed decision regarding whether the study is of value to *us*.

THE 'CRITICAL' IN CRITICAL APPRAISAL

The 'critical' element is perhaps too often considered the emphasis of critical appraisal, with many setting out to 'trash' research (Greenhalgh 2006). The reality is that both strengths and weaknesses should be identified and weighed up to determine whether, overall, the results are useful. Hill and Spittlehouse (2001) acknowledge that most research is not perfect, but emphasize that although critical appraisal is not an exact science, it can help us determine if a piece of research is *good enough* to be used to inform our practice. Landorf and Keenan (2000) summarized this point by stating that the focus should not only be on strengths and weaknesses, but also on their contribution to our understanding of the topic. They claim that most research, if carefully planned, will contribute to our knowledge in some way, and also assert that it is inappropriate to dismiss a research article on the basis of small flaws when the research base, taken as a whole, does not support this. Therefore, the challenge of critical appraisal is not to try to find flaws that let us dismiss the research out of hand: it is to draw a balanced conclusion based on careful consideration of strengths and weaknesses. The process demands objectivity to permit a balanced conclusion to be drawn, and although disadvantages include an increased effort during the original development of the techniques, considerable advantages are at stake (Box 5.1).

Box 5.1 The pros and cons of critical appraisal in practice (Hill & Spittlehouse 2001)

Pros of critical appraisal
- Critical appraisal provides a systematic way of assessing the validity, results and usefulness of published research papers.
- Critical appraisal can help close the gap between research and practice and, as such, makes an essential contribution to improving healthcare.
- Critical appraisal encourages objective assessment of the usefulness of information. Critical appraisal skills are applied to published research, but all evidence should be appraised to weigh up its usefulness.
- Critical appraisal skills are not difficult to develop. Critical appraisal is a common-sense approach to reading, and user-friendly tools are available to help anyone develop these skills.

Cons of critical appraisal
- The process can be time-consuming initially, although with time it becomes second nature.
- It does not always provide the 'easy answer' or the answer hoped for: it may actually highlight that a favoured intervention is, in fact, ineffective.
- It can be discouraging if it highlights a lack of good-quality evidence, and it may take determination to persist with an area of interest when access to good research in the area is limited.

CRITICAL APPRAISAL AND VALIDITY

At the start of this chapter we asserted that critical appraisal is essentially a 'quality and suitability' analysis. In technical terms these issues relate to *validity*. The concept of validity is important as this theme runs all the way through the process of critical appraisal. The basic definition of validity relates to the extent to which a measurement represents a true value – asking if a measurement instrument is capable of correctly measuring the variable of interest (Vetter & Matthews 1999). Whilst this definition is appropriate when considering a measurement tool, a wider application of the concept is required when asking: 'Is this research valid?' A valid research study will have employed not only an accurate measurement technique, but will also have employed a suitable research design for the question being investigated, recruited a well-defined group of subjects, appropriately analysed the results obtained and drawn appropriate conclusions. This means that the results will have meaning: we can relate them to a defined population, can be confident that the measurements obtained are accurate and that the research design has provided information relevant to the question that was asked. When we are confident that these dimensions of the research were valid, we can make an informed judgement about whether we can justifiably use the research to inform the way we treat our patients.

The application of the concept of validity to a series of issues within a piece of research is recognized in the way the term is defined. We need to understand a little about the concepts involved in preparation for tackling the question: 'Is this research valid?' The reality is that it is difficult to provide a simple yes/no answer to this question, because whilst most research will have attained an acceptable level of validity in some ways, it may have missed the mark in others. Validity, therefore, needs to be considered on different levels and should be regarded as a multi-dimensional concept.

The multiple dimensions of 'validity' can be illustrated by considering the measurement tool used in any study. If it appears to be appropriate to the question being investigated – for example, through the use of an appropriate method, suitable subjects and accurate measurement techniques – it can be said to have *face* validity: on the face of it the measurement tool appears appropriate. However, if closer examination of the measurement technique reveals that it oversimplifies the variable being measured, then *content* validity is compromised. This means that the separate dimensions of the variable being measured are inadequately represented. For example, if we are measuring foot pain we could use a visual analogue scale which scores pain on a scale between 1 and 10. However, it would be more appropriate to use the Rowan foot pain assessment questionnaire (Rowan 2001) which considers sensory (what the patient feels), cognitive (how the pain makes the patient think) and affective dimensions of pain (how the pain causes the patient to change their behaviour), as it considers more dimensions of the pain experience. This means that it has greater content validity. If the questionnaire score accurately reflects the true level of pain experienced by the patient then this would infer *criterion* validity, whilst its ability to predict a clinically important outcome relates to *construct* validity. Therefore, if the Rowan pain score accurately predicted a reduced functional capacity, it could be said to have construct validity. Validity can be complex, but the message is that we should be more convinced by the results of a study, and therefore be more likely to use them, if validity is satisfied on various levels as opposed to just one. The core dimensions of validity are summarized in Box 5.2.

Box 5.2 Validity and some core dimensions (Gomm et al 2000)

Validity

Technically, validity is defined as the extent to which a measurement tool measures what it claims to. However, in relation to a research study, validity relates to the adequacy of the research design to achieve the original aim. Thus, validity is determined by a series of factors involved in research design, from the characteristics and inclusion criteria for the subjects recruited, to the time period over which the study was conducted and the duration of the follow-up period. Validity is a complex construct, and as such we will encounter a variety of different 'types' of validity referred to in the literature. Several core dimensions of validity are as follows:

- *Face validity*: The apparent adequacy of the measurement tool on first inspection, in relation to what is being measured. If the tool seems to fit the bill, then it appears, on the face of it, to be valid.
- *Content validity*: Are the separate dimensions of the variable being measured represented in the measurement tool? If there are a number of dimensions to a particular variable, and the tool examines each one, then the content is judged valid.
- *Criterion validity*: If the results obtained by a measurement tool are compared with an external gold standard technique, and there is a close correlation between the two instruments, then the measurement tool can be said to have criterion validity.
- *Construct validity*: Refers to the correlation between an instrument's score and clinically important outcomes such as prognosis.

Ultimately, we read research to influence how *we* practice: this means that we must reference our appraisal to *our* patients in *our* clinical environment. This is in contrast to a journal's peer-review process, which has no knowledge of our situation and so focuses on general methodological or analytical errors. It cannot possibly determine the relevance of the study to *our* patients, even if the study was of high quality. Because we have responsibility for treating our patients, it therefore falls to us to critically evaluate research to determine:

- the validity of the research (which tells us if the results are to be believed)
- the application of the results to our practice (which tells us if the results of the research can be applied to our patients).

It is important to appreciate that a research study cannot be applicable to our patients if it is not valid, but that a study that is valid need not be applicable to our patients. The ability to relate the results of a study to other patients is termed *external* validity (relating to the application of the results to subjects or patients *external to*, or outside, the study subjects).

THE TENSION BETWEEN CRITICAL APPRAISAL AND RESEARCH DESIGN

In Chapter 2 the term 'research skills' was explained in terms of the differing knowledge requirements of active researchers and practising clinicians. The process of evidence-based practice was suggested to be vitally important to all practising healthcare professionals, whilst traditional research methods were suggested to be more important for active researchers. This led to the conclusion that the knowledge requirements of the two groups could be separated out somewhat. Whilst this is true to a certain extent, it is not quite so simple. This is because knowledge of research skills will naturally improve our understanding of how to conduct research, and vice versa: involvement in active research will help us to understand the characteristics of good-quality research, which, in turn, will allow us to perform a more effective critical appraisal. Therefore, it is not possible to divorce skills of research design and methods from skills of critical appraisal.

The result of the relationship between research skills and research methods is that there is tension between the two whereby we cannot develop knowledge in relation to one without simultaneously developing knowledge of the other. This may make it seem that undertaking a critical appraisal is a difficult task that requires specialist knowledge of research methods. Whilst it is certainly true that complex research studies require substantial knowledge and experience to appraise, and detailed knowledge of methods and statistics will help us appraise every last detail of even more modest research, help is at hand for the novice in the form of critical appraisal 'systems' or 'tools'. These guides to the process are invaluable, because they help us ask the right questions at the right time.

KEY CONCEPT

The language of research

To perform a critical appraisal we must get to grips with the language of research. A variety of terms are used in the research literature, and although some may be familiar, we must be sure that we have an accurate understanding of their meaning within research. It is therefore vital to have a glossary of terms, a dictionary or a research textbook to hand to provide definitions of terms encountered.

CRITICAL APPRAISAL TOOLS AND THEIR ROLE

Critical appraisal tools range from chapters in research texts which provide an overview of the major issues that require consideration, to specialist books such as *The Pocket Guide to Critical Appraisal* (Crombie 1996) which is dedicated to the topic. A useful development has been the formulation of a number of more focused tools, such as the Critical Appraisal Skills Programme (CASP) and the CONSORT statement, which provide checklists that are directed at particular types of study.

The adoption of a formal critical appraisal tool is associated with various advantages. This was demonstrated in a study that sought to determine whether a group of general practitioners using a formal appraisal system were more likely to agree with an expert appraisal than a group using their own approach (MacAuley et al 1998). The system used was named *READER* after the issues covered: *Relevance* to practice (Is it relevant to me?), *Education* (Will it influence my practice?), *Applicability* (Is it possible to do what is suggested?), *Discrimination* (methodological quality) and *overall Evaluation* (previous categories summed), with each category scored using a simple scale. Results revealed the system to be accurate and repeatable, with those utilizing the system being more critical in their reading and acknowledging that they were more likely to maintain this in future. Although we must not be discouraged from asking our own questions as they arise when we read a study (which are likely to be important as they are generated in context), the use of a formal system provides a good framework from which to develop our appraisal.

KEY CONCEPT

Critical appraisal tools

A critical appraisal tool may also be referred to as an 'instrument' or 'system'. In their purest form these tools comprise a checklist of questions which focus our attention on a series of critical issues that contribute to the overall validity of the research. However, there are also chapters in research texts and dedicated books that help us to understand the issues involved and formulate an approach to the task.

To be suitably armed to tackle the appraisal of a range of research reports we need to be familiar with a range of the available tools. This will also help us to develop our appraisal of any particular study appropriately, as we bring in additional questions to probe further where we see the need. Each tool adopts a slightly different approach, and using a variety of tools will encourage the development of the depth and breadth of knowledge that is required to confidently appraise the research with which we are routinely faced. Firstly, an overview of the process can be found in the critical appraisal chapters of modern research methods texts. Background information and general concepts are presented in a discursive manner which underpins the basic question lists that are often provided. These lists are similar to the preliminary questions presented in specialized texts, which are the second category of appraisal tool available. Specialist texts help us consolidate and develop our knowledge by providing greater background detail and more sophisticated explanations of key issues, together with more detailed question lists that delve deeper into methods and results sections. These equip us to use the final category of resource – checklists – which provide lists of focused questions but limited accompanying information on their rationale and implications.

A BASIC APPROACH TO CRITICAL APPRAISAL: THE IMRAD SYSTEM

A useful place to begin when developing skills of critical appraisal is with consideration of the information that should be provided within the research report. One such system is *IMRAD*, which considers the *Introduction, Method, Results* and *Discussion* sections in turn to determine if they provide the appropriate information. This seems a useful place to begin when it is considered that most papers appearing in medical journals are presented in this format (Greenhalgh 2000). This approach forms the basis of that described in chapters in general research texts (e.g. Polgar & Thomas 2000) which aim to provide an introduction to the process, and also in the introductory chapters of specialist textbooks. For example, the second chapter of Crombie's (1996) *Pocket Guide to Critical Appraisal* proposes six questions designed to elicit the important information that should be provided in each section (Box 5.3).

Box 5.3 Questions to ask when reading a paper (Crombie 1996)

'Preliminary questions' suggested by Crombie to elicit the information that each section contains. This approach mirrors IMRAD.

- Is it of interest?   (*Introduction*)
- Why was it done?   (*Introduction*)
- How was it done?   (*Method*)
- What has it found?   (*Results*)
- What are the implications?   (*Discussion*)
- What else is of interest?

By their very nature, research reports tend to focus on specialist areas of study and, as such, may use complex language. However, they should not be inaccessible because of this, and it should be possible to glean a core set of details from each section. If the language is overly complex, then it may very well be that the authors are hiding something behind this façade of complexity: put simply, we are looking for clarity in the expression of this information with the objectivity of *The Independent* (a balanced, objective UK newspaper), but in the writing style of *The Sun* (a tabloid UK newspaper written in a simpler style).

EXERCISE

IMRAD appraisal involves assessment of the main sections of the research report. Think about the headings *Introduction, Method, Results* and *Discussion* and write down some notes on what you think is the purpose of each section. Explain your answer.

INTRODUCTION

The introduction sets the scene for the research report and, as such, should provide the reader with clear information regarding the background to the issue. Its importance should be explained (e.g. in terms of the economic or psychosocial costs associated with the problem) to make it clear why the issue deserves attention. The 'state of the art' should be conveyed succinctly with an emphasis on both what is known and what is not yet known. Identifying what is not known is vital, as these are the areas requiring further research. However, don't expect a comprehensive literature review: the word limit on research reports is finite, with most journals setting a limit of between 2000 and 4000 words for original research articles. Nevertheless, a clear and logical background should be provided and the rationale behind and purpose of the study should be crystal clear.

Basic appraisal of the introduction

The introduction is all about *justifying the research* investigation and demonstrating how it fits with existing knowledge. As such, several questions should be asked:

- Is the purpose of the study clearly stated?
- Is the importance of the proposed study made clear?
- Who will the research benefit/what are the benefits?
- How does the study complement existing research?

If these questions can be clearly answered, then the introduction has justified the proposed investigation. Conversely, if the answers are unclear, or cannot be discerned, it is difficult to carry on with the appraisal. Just think how difficult it will be to appraise the method if you are not clear on the question it is trying to answer.

METHOD

The method should provide details of exactly *how* the study was performed. It is the most important section of a research report, as it is the major determinant of validity. If the method is unclear, ambiguous, sloppy or is flawed in any way, the quality of the data gathered will be compromised. Not all flaws will have serious consequences, however, and the challenge becomes balancing each flaw against its influence on the results obtained. Whilst some flaws are fatal, others exert a more minor influence, and we must determine which category a flaw falls into before rejecting the paper out of hand.

CLINICAL TIP

Approaching an IMRAD appraisal

The IMRAD approach focuses on each section of the research report. Summarizing your answers to the main questions relating to each section will quickly reveal whether adequate information has been provided. If you cannot easily summarize a section, then it is likely that important information is missing or is provided in overly complex language.

The method can be evaluated on two levels: a basic level, addressed by an IMRAD appraisal involving assessment of the 'completeness' of the information provided, and a more advanced level that considers the suitability and execution of the research design chosen.

Firstly, we are interested in the detail that has been provided explaining how the study was done. There should be sufficient detail to allow the study to be repeated, and information on the sample, the apparatus used and the protocol followed should be provided. Often it is not practical to provide full details of every aspect of the method within the constraints of a published article with a limited word count. It is therefore common to include references to other research papers where the method is described in detail. In fact, the validity of a paper is enhanced if the authors can refer the reader to more extensive accounts of how a particular measurement technique or data collection protocol was developed and validated. This shows that an accepted technique has been employed. After reading the methods section we should feel that we have sufficient information to repeat the study.

Secondly, the methods section can be evaluated in terms of the suitability of the research design used and the way in which that design was executed. This demands an understanding of the available research designs and the types of question they were designed to tackle. An overview of the broad fields of research employed in healthcare was provided by Greenhalgh (2006), and this serves as a useful introduction to the basic categories of research and the questions they are designed to investigate (Box 5.4). Advanced critical appraisal demands greater knowledge of individual research designs and their conduct.

Box 5.4 Broad fields of research (after Greenhalgh 2006)

- *Cause*: Investigates the suspected substances, exposures or behaviours linked to the development of a disease. Commonly uses case-control or cohort designs.
- *Screening*: Aims to evaluate the likely impact of tests which can be administered to large populations and which identify disease in the early stages of development, prior to clinical signs and symptoms developing. Uses cross-sectional designs.
- *Therapy*: Evaluates the efficacy of any interventions used by healthcare professionals, ranging from drug treatment to surgical and non-surgical interventions, and systems of service delivery. Favoured design is the randomized controlled trial.
- *Diagnosis*: Studies evaluating the validity and reliability of diagnostic tests. This involves the investigation of accuracy by calculating the rate of false positives and false negatives associated with the test. Also evaluates reliability – consistency between repeated tests. Cross-sectional design used.
- *Prognosis*: Evaluation of outcomes over various lengths of time of patients with specific diseases. Longitudinal study design used.
- *Psychometric*: Investigation of attitudes, beliefs or preferences. In healthcare this could be about service organization, the effects of a disease or its treatment, and the needs of patients with a particular disease.

Basic appraisal of the method

Basic appraisal of the method focuses on describing what was actually done. Key issues to consider include the following:

- What was done?
- To whom was it done, and what is important, special or unique about that group of individuals? Are they representative of a larger population?
- Was appropriate data recorded – in terms of participant characteristics and study measurements?
- How exactly were the data collected, and what equipment was used?

After reading the method you should have a clear idea of how to carry out the data collection yourself. If you are not sure of exactly what was done, then the methods section has not done its job. This makes it difficult to judge validity and, as such, prevents the use of the results to inform practice.

RESULTS

The results section is perhaps the most daunting section of a research report for the novice. However, the associated angst can be reduced if the results are evaluated in the context of the method: if we know the measurement tool that was used and the measurements that this tool yields, then we should be curious about the measurements that were obtained. Therefore, the reader should have an *information requirement* and should look for that information in the results section.

Similar to the method, the results section should be descriptive, in that it should describe important characteristics of the subjects that took part in the study and the measurements gathered from them. In fact, *descriptive statistics* is a term used to describe one type of data provided in the results. These numbers are essentially summary details of the subjects or the scores generated using the data collection technique. This is easily illustrated using the example of a lecture room full of students. We can record measurements related to a variety of different factors to describe such a group. For example, we could measure IQ, ethnic origin, eye colour, hair colour, body mass index, country of origin, distance travelled to get to the lecture or even criminal convictions. Absolutely *any* characteristic can be measured and summarized, and when we do this we are describing the subjects. Descriptive statistics summarize information for practical reasons. If we have a group of 50 students it would be difficult to look at 50 individual numbers and attach any meaning to them. However, if we can summarize these 50 scores by calculating an average then we immediately have a useful idea of the measures within the group. This is all descriptive statistics are doing – summarizing lots of pieces of information to produce an overall picture.

A study will often involve comparison of information gathered from multiple groups. If group A has an average IQ of 118, group B has an average of 100 and group C has an average of 104, it is clear that the IQ levels are different between the three groups. Clearly the differences between 100 and 118, and 104 and 118 are fairly large, and likely to indicate disparity between the groups. However, the difference between 100 and 104 is small and, as such, it may be difficult to judge if this difference reflects an important variation. This is where the second type of statistics comes in – inferential statistics. Briefly, this type of statistic estimates the likelihood that two groups of scores came from the same population. Inferential statistics will be discussed more fully in Chapter 6.

Basic appraisal of the results

Getting to grips with the results requires us to ask several questions regarding the data that were collected:

- How were the subjects described?
  - What measurements were recorded and what were the units of measurement?
- Were the subjects described in a meaningful way?
  - For example, their age, sex, height, weight, socioeconomic group. The only rules governing the way in which study subjects should be described is that it must be important to the study being conducted.
- Were the study measurements described in a straightforward way?
  - Think about the results. If you are not happy with the information provided because it prevents you from understanding the study completely, then comment on it. If you think that some important information should be provided, and can justify why, this detracts from the study as it compromises your understanding.
- Do the numbers add up?
  - The numbers provided in the results section should make sense, i.e. they should be clear, unambiguous and make sense. A little mental arithmetic can help you determine if the data provided actually make sense. For example, numbers 8, 10, 12, 10 and 12 cannot possibly have an average of 6 or 12. Looking at the results on even such a simple level can enhance understanding.
- Do the tables and graphs help you understand the data?
  - Tables and graphs should not be provided just because every results section should have at least one of each. They are included to provide important information that will *enhance the reader's understanding*. Furthermore, there should always be reference to tables and graphs in the text, i.e. they should be clearly anchored to the text. There should also be a legend describing what they are illustrating and their purpose, so that they can 'stand alone', i.e. they can be understood without reading the entire results section.

By the end of the results section you should be able to write some brief notes stating what the results were. Further, you should be able to describe the characteristics of the study population. If you can't, then either insufficient information has been provided or the section is overly complex.

DISCUSSION

The discussion is where the results are put into context. This is done in two ways:

1. The validity of the results is considered by carefully weighing up the strengths and weaknesses of the method by which they were obtained. This tells us if we can consider them accurate.

2. The importance of the results to knowledge and understanding of the subject is discussed by linking back to key concepts presented in the introduction. This tells us to whom and to what situations we can apply the results.

Our appraisal of these elements of the study tells us firstly if the results are to be believed, and secondly it tells us that if they are to be believed, then this is what they mean.

Basic appraisal of the discussion

The focus of the discussion should be on the appropriate interpretation of the results. Therefore, several questions are key:

- Are sources of error identified, and are the implications of these potential errors considered?
- Are any key sources of error unidentified?

KEY CONCEPT

Homogeneity and heterogeneity

Subjects in a study sample can be described as homogeneous if they are similar – for example, all children, all young adults, all middle-aged or elderly, or all the same sex, or height, or weight. Heterogeneity means that they are different. For example, they range in age from 12 to 65 years, are male and female, are underweight, optimal weight or overweight, or all take a range of different medications.

We want subjects to be the 'same' in a study. If a study group is highly variable, then the true effect that could be expected in any particular patient becomes difficult to predict.

However, this issue is a double-edged sword. A homogeneous study sample means that the study recruited patients who are unlikely to be encountered in clinical practice – where large differences in many variables are routinely encountered.

A trial which recruits a homogeneous sample can therefore be applauded for the strength of evidence it provides, but criticized for failing to reflect real life.

Adopting the IMRAD approach provides a useful insight into the thought that has gone into the development of the research question, the design and the conduct of the research. However, this represents an introductory appraisal, and a more detailed analysis of the methods and results sections is required. Whilst the methods section will be considered further here, the results will be considered in Chapter 6 which discusses research design.

UPPING THE ANTE: UNDERSTANDING THE RESEARCH METHOD

The method is a vital part of every research report. If it is well designed it will yield valid results that can be used to inform practice. However, if it is poorly designed it may be flawed in such a way that it will not yield valid results and so should not be used to inform practice. Therefore, when developing skills in critical appraisal, this section warrants greater attention than any other. Two issues must be addressed:

1. the suitability of the research method for the question under investigation
2. if the research method was suitable for the question being asked, the rigour with which that design was applied.

ASSESSING THE SUITABILITY OF THE RESEARCH DESIGN

Various research methods are available, with each designed to investigate specific questions. The major research designs used in health research have been organized into a 'hierarchy of evidence' (Greenhalgh 2000) (Fig. 5.1), which ranks the designs in terms of the strength of evidence each provides regarding the effectiveness of interventions.

It is important to remember that the hierarchy of evidence is organized in terms of the evidence each design provides in relation to the analysis of *treatments*. The misinterpretation of the hierarchy of evidence has resulted in a common misconception that randomized controlled trials are the gold standard study design. However, this ignores the context in which the hierarchy was formulated, i.e. in relation to the analysis of treatments (Black 1998, Miettinen 1998, Tanenbaum 1999). As a simple literature review of

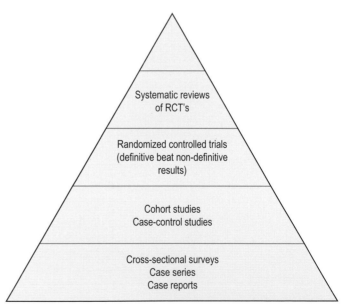

Figure 5.1 The hierarchy of evidence, which ranks common study designs according to the strength of evidence they provide regarding the analysis of treatments. Systematic reviews are a secondary research design in that they review a series of original studies, whilst all other designs are primary, original studies. The pyramid shows systematic reviews at the pinnacle of the hierarchy, whilst case reports lie at the bottom.

CLINICAL TIP

The hierarchy of evidence

This popular concept ranks common designs according to the value of the information they can produce regarding effective treatments. However, only the randomized controlled trial is designed to investigate this issue and, as such, we should not use this concept to judge the value of a design.

any condition will reveal, research is not solely concerned with the analysis of treatments. Often it will evaluate the rate of occurrence of a condition (e.g. diabetes) or a health behaviour (e.g. eating junk food or smoking), or will aim to identify who gets a condition, what causes it or why the public adopt the health behaviours they do (e.g. why do people smoke?). The hierarchy of evidence also neglects to consider the role of qualitative research techniques. These designs can help yield information on, for example, how patients feel about their health or why they adopt particular health behaviours. To develop a comprehensive understanding of a subject, we need information from various sources and, as such, it is more appropriate to think of each research design not as a hierarchy in which one design is superior to all others, but as a jigsaw where each design is a piece which contributes to a complete understanding of a subject (Fig. 5.2).

A simple awareness of the common designs, the information they provide and the way they interact, can be developed by considering this example:

Case studies provide rapid information on an interesting/unique/ important issue in the context of a single patient encounter...In *cross-sectional surveys* a sample of subjects is interviewed, examined or otherwise studied to gain answers to a specific clinical question, for example, relating to how widespread our initial observation may be....*Case control studies* then recruit 'control' subjects to provide information on the value of what we observed in our case...*Cohort studies* follow subjects who are normal to see who develops the disease with time in relation to the factors to which they are exposed. A *randomized controlled trial* may then be used to evaluate the interventions. When we have lots of randomized controlled trials we can then systematically review them to determine the consistency of the evidence from randomized controlled trials to inform practice.

The essence of... case studies

Case studies are regarded as the weakest form of evidence. This is because they focus on only one subject and, as such, may represent the exception to the rule. They should not focus on run of the mill matters – they identify a

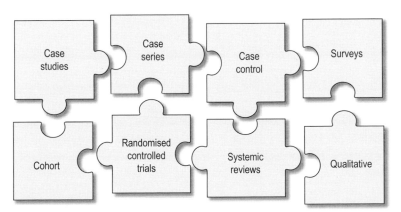

Figure 5.2 The various research designs complement each other to provide a clear and comprehensive 'picture' of the issue.

unique dimension to a case to draw it to their colleagues' attention. They may focus on diagnostic techniques, an unusual cause or presentation of a problem, or a novel treatment. The important aspect of a case study is that it should present something unique. Case studies are often abused by students who simply describe a routine presentation of a routine problem!

The essence of...cross-sectional surveys

Surveys are investigations that gather measurements from populations to describe specific characteristics. We probably all have experience of surveys – it is likely that most of us have been stopped in the street at some point and asked our opinion on a specific issue, or have received a consumer household survey in the post. Polgar and Thomas (2000) state that surveys are commonly used for three purposes in health research:

- establishing the attitudes, opinions or beliefs of people concerning health-related matters, e.g. attitudes to exercise or diet
- studying health-related characteristics in populations, e.g. blood pressure, obesity, blood glucose level
- gathering demographic information, e.g. age, socioeconomic status, income, occupation. (A government census is an important survey that examines demographic information on a population.)

Surveys make a unique contribution to our understanding of the distribution of characteristics in the population, and help us understand how people feel about certain issues.

The essence of...case-control studies

Case-control studies involve the recruitment of a group of cases (individuals with a specific disease) and a group of controls (a group of individuals without the disease) for comparison purposes. The concept behind this design is that differences in the characteristics of the groups may reveal information regarding the cause of the disease. For example, if we recruit a group of individuals with lung cancer and a group without, we may identify that they differ in terms of smoking behaviour. This design cannot prove that smoking causes lung cancer – it can only provide information suggesting that there may be a link. This concept is illustrated by considering early research concerning smoking, which also suggested that alcohol intake was important. This finding was related to the association between smoking and drinking, which obscured the role of the individual factors. In this example alcohol intake was a confounding factor. Bland (2000) defined confounding as any factor that unintentionally influences a study to distort conclusions. In the scenario above, alcohol acted to confound the relationship between smoking and lung cancer.

The essence of...cohort studies

Cohort studies involve the monitoring of a group of individuals to see what happens to them over time and in relation to exposure to a particular variable(s). The concept is illustrated below. Cohort studies are characterized by their organization of individuals, at the start of the study, into groups based on their exposure to a defined factor(s). The subjects are then followed over time to determine the influence of the exposure on the onset of particular diseases. They do not need to focus on disease – they may consider protective effects. For example, by recruiting women taking hormone replacement therapy and those who do not, the protection provided by this intervention to cardiovascular events or osteoporotic fractures can be evaluated.

Illustration of a cohort study

Two populations are defined in terms of their exposure to a variable of interest, and are followed up over a period of time, which can be years, to determine what happens to the members of each group.

| Exposed | | Non-exposed | |
| Develop disease | Don't develop disease | Develop disease | Don't develop disease |

Perhaps the most famous cohort study is the Framingham study, designed to examine the role of various factors perceived to be related to the development of cardiovascular disease. Framingham is a town on the east coast of America with a population of ~30 000. Out of this population, 5127 men and women between 30 and 62 years of age entered the study at its inception in 1948. Various 'exposures', including smoking, obesity, blood pressure, cholesterol and physical activity, were monitored. Heart problems were tracked by examining the participants every 2 years and by daily monitoring of admissions to the only hospital in the town. The study was designed to run for 20 years, but this follow-up period was exceeded, with a 40-year update appearing in 1990 (Kannel 1990). The exposures that were examined in this study may seem a strange choice because of what we now know, but our understanding of these factors actually came from Framingham.

An important feature of both cohort and case-control studies is that they recognize that some of those who are not exposed to the variable we are interested in may still develop the disease, i.e. non-smokers may develop lung cancer. However, it is reasonable to expect that more smokers will develop lung cancer than non-smokers. The use of a comparison group, who are not exposed to the exposure of interest, is therefore vital, and allows the *attributable proportion* to be calculated. This provides an estimate of the number of people developing the disease due to the exposure of interest and an insight into the number of events that may be prevented by eliminating exposure to that factor (Gordis 2004).

The essence of...randomized controlled trials

RCTs represent the 'gold standard' study design for assessing the effectiveness of treatments. The design is based on the premise that:

1. some people will improve despite the treatment they are given, not because of it
2. it is difficult (impossible?) to account for all the characteristics of subjects that may influence the outcome of a study.

Comparing the treatment of interest with no treatment, a placebo (physiologically inactive) treatment or the best currently available treatment

Library
Knowledge Spa
Royal Cornwall Hospital
Treliske
Truro. TR1 3HD

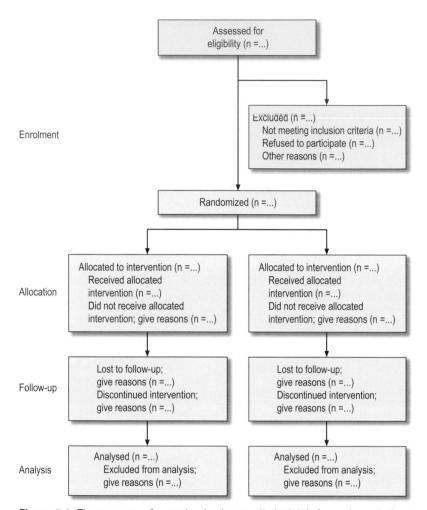

Figure 5.3 The progress of a randomized controlled trial. Information relating to each stage should be provided (after Moher et al 2001).

tackles the first scenario. The second scenario is tackled by randomly allocating a group of eligible participants to receive any of the options that are available in the trial. This theoretically distributes a whole host of undefined characteristics between the groups to minimize the possibility of them influencing the outcome of the study.

The design of an RCT is often summarized in diagrammatic form (Moher et al 2001), and this is a useful method of illustrating the key features (Fig. 5.3). Firstly, a suitable population is selected, from which a suitable sample is obtained. As each subject must have an equal chance of receiving either treatment, a randomization procedure must be employed to achieve this. Ideally, subjects should be 'blinded' to the group they are in, so that they do not know which treatment they are receiving. Although it is not always possible, the researcher should also be unaware of which subjects are receiving which treatments. This reduces the likelihood of the results being unfairly influenced by researcher or subject expectations (Vetter & Matthews 1999).

The RCT design can be illustrated using the example of Moseley et al (2002), which Gordis (2004) described as 'beautifully conducted'. This study sought to investigate the true value of knee arthroscopy for osteoarthritis – a common procedure – the effectiveness of which seemed to be related more to patient expectations than to the actual procedure. The study recruited 180 subjects who were randomly allocated to receive arthroscopic debridement, a simple washout or a sham procedure involving a skin incision without insertion of the arthroscope, but with 'simulated' surgery. Subjects were followed up for 2 years, with pain and function among the outcomes considered. Over the 2-year follow-up period, neither the arthroscopic debridement nor the washout group demonstrated significantly better outcomes than the sham surgery group. The authors concluded that surgery was no better than a placebo. As well as illustrating the concept of the RCT, this study highlights the power of the placebo effect.

The essence of...systematic reviews

Systematic reviews attempt to tackle the controversy that exists where several treatments are available for a particular disorder but the most effective one is unknown. They sit at the top of the hierarchy of literature because they are a secondary research design, as opposed to all the others which are termed *primary* research. Whilst a primary research report provides details of a single piece of research, secondary research tries to find all of the trials that have been conducted on a well-defined issue. It then appraises these *systematically* using a criterion-based marking system to produce a quality score for each article. An example of a quality rating system is the CONSORT statement (Consolidated Standards for Reporting Trials) which focuses on clinical trials (Moher et al 2001). A general conclusion is then drawn by considering the 'level of evidence' that the literature provides. The concept of 'levels of evidence' adheres to the concept of the hierarchy of literature by ranking studies according to the methodology employed (Table 5.1). A general conclusion on the 'grade of recommendation' that can be applied is then drawn (Table 5.2). However, systematic reviews almost always conclude that more primary research of a higher quality is required.

ASSESSING THE RIGOUR WITH WHICH THE RESEARCH DESIGN WAS APPLIED

After considering the suitability of the research design and the general appropriateness of the information provided in the main sections of the report, we can turn our attention to the way that the design was executed. Each design is capable of enhancing our understanding but only if it was performed appropriately. Each research design is characterized by the use of unique methodological 'devices' which ensure the quality of the resulting information; because of this, checklists have been presented for each of the main types of design (CASP 2006, Crombie 1996). However, as these specific checklists share some general characteristics, we propose the division of questions in three categories:

1. a clear research question should be provided and the design adopted by the study should be appropriate for tackling this question

Table 5.1 Levels of evidence* (Oxford Centre for Evidance-based Medicine 2001)

Level	Study design
1a	A convincing systematic review (i.e. that identified consistency between multiple studies)
1b	An individual RCT that identifies a clear effect
1c	A special category reserved for interventions where limited information is available, but where patient survival is improved with the treatment in question
2a	A systematic review with conflicting/inconsistent findings
2b	An individual cohort study or low quality RCT
2c	Ecological studies (evaluation of group characteristics, e.g. association between fat intake and breast cancer, using information from a series of countries)
3a	A systematic review of case-control studies
3b	An individual case-control study
4	A case series or poor quality cohort/case-control study
5	Expert opinion, with explicit critical appraisal

* A systematic review considers the literature and ranks each study according to the strength of evidence it provides.

Table 5.2 Grades of recommendation* (Oxford Centre for Evidence-based Medicine 2001)

Grade	Nature of evidence
A	Consistent level 1 studies
B	Consistent level 2 or 3 studies *or* extrapolations from level 1 studies
C	Level 4 studies *or* extrapolations from level 2 or 3 studies
D	Level 5 studies *or* troublingly inconsistent studies of any level

*How to rate the strength of evidence concerning clinical practices. We want our practice to be based on the highest grade of recommendation.

2. questions relating to sample selection, the measurement techniques employed and potential elements of bias, chance and confounding should be posed
3. the 'believability' of the results and their local application should be considered.

To consider the rigour with which the design was executed, it is the questions relating to the second category that are more important. Regardless of the design, methodological issues relate to sample selection, measurement techniques and the steps taken to minimize the play of bias, chance and confounding.

Issue 1: Is the sample, and the population from which they are drawn, well defined?

A sample must be carefully chosen so that they are truly representative of the population from which they were drawn. A useful analogy is to consider a cake-eating competition. A judge in such a competition would not eat every last piece of every cake, but would instead eat a single piece of each cake. This piece would not be a small crumb, but nor would it need to be a complete portion – it would perhaps be a few mouthfuls. A judgement would then be made based on the assumption that the sample was representative of the rest of the cake. A study sample is selected on the same principle. If we are interested in a specific population we do not need to assess every single member of that population – we need to select a number of the population who are representative. This leads us to ask ourselves if it is clear to whom the results can be applied. If the study was conducted on a clearly defined group we can answer this question, but if the sample was heterogeneous (mixed), then it is difficult to determine exactly to whom the results can confidently be applied. This concept can also be applied to systematic reviews, where the sample is a series of research papers. Providing information on how these were selected is just as vital for this design as is the selection of subjects.

Issue 2: Are the variables measured in the study well defined and measured using an accepted, accurate technique?

Every study involves measurement. It may be the number of people with a disease, an attitude or opinion or belief, or a measurement of a biological variable such as blood pressure or joint range of motion. Whenever any variable is measured, at any stage of a study, it is vital that an accepted technique is adopted for doing so. The quality of the results obtained is determined by the accuracy of the measurement technique. We should look for clear information on precisely what was measured and the measurement technique used. Furthermore, it is entirely reasonable to expect the study to provide a justification for the use of this technique. Remember that if the measurements upon which the results are based are flawed, then the results are seriously – perhaps even fatally – flawed. Every time a measurement is taken, the same protocol and technique should be used; in the case-control design, this means that both groups should be measured in exactly the same way. In cohort studies, which can involve repeated measurements over many years, it is vital that the same technique is used every time that measurement is recorded. The potential consequence of using different techniques is that successive measurements may then fail to reflect a true change in the variable of interest, and instead reflect a change in the measurement technique. This issue is critical in research, and the all-important concepts of measurement validity and reliability will be considered in some detail in Chapter 6.

Issue 3: Can any elements of bias, chance or confounding be identified that could influence the results?

Bias relates to any factor which erroneously influences the conclusions about groups and distorts comparisons (Greenhalgh 2006). Chance refers to exactly what it says: an association that is identified purely by luck, when in actual fact no such association exists. Confounding was described by Vetter and Matthews (1999) as variables that are associated with both the disease and the suspected causative factor which indicate a relationship when one does not, in fact, exist. For example, because many years ago people went to the pub to drink and smoke, drinking appeared to be related to lung cancer. It is not, of course, but because many people who smoke drink alcohol, it acted as a confounding factor.

Selecting an appropriate sample size helps to reduce the likelihood of these factors exerting a significant influence on results. However, various pragmatic steps can also be taken to minimize the play of these factors as exemplified in the randomized controlled trial design.

The RCT design is illustrated in Figure 5.3. It begins with recruitment of all patients eligible for treatment based on explicit inclusion–exclusion criteria. A *randomization* procedure is then used to randomly allocate eligible subjects to receive one of two (or even more) treatments. The allocation of subjects to groups should be, if possible and ethical, *double-blind*. This means that neither the patient nor the researcher knows which treatment any participant received: they are simply taking treatment 'A' or 'B'. However, on occasion, it may only be possible for the study to be single-blind, as the patient needs to know which treatment they are receiving.

Issue 4: Is every subject recruited accounted for at the end of the study?

Information on follow-up is vital as it helps us put the results in context, otherwise we make assumptions. For example, if an RCT approached 500 potential subjects, but managed to recruit only 100 of these, of whom a further 35 dropped out, this is important information and we should ask ourselves why this happened. Were there untoward events, was the intervention unacceptable or did the subjects find the study unpalatable? If the information is provided we can draw conclusions, but if it is not provided then we simply do not know, and this makes it difficult to draw conclusions confidently. Therefore, subject follow-up, and details of any subject who dropped out together with the reasons, should be provided.

After considering the rigour with which the method was applied, we are ready to move on to consideration of the results and their 'local' application. However, this information is best considered in a more general discussion of research methods, which is provided in Chapter 6.

CASE STUDY REVISITED

The decision on whether to use the results obtained by a study is related to the quality of the design employed, and so a critical appraisal is warranted. What follows is a focused critique of some of the main factors in a study carried out by Riddle et al (2003).

Case-control studies are a design that focuses on identifying factors that could be associated with a disease. As the aim of this study is clearly stated as being 'to determine whether risk factors for plantar fasciitis could be identified', the case-control design seems appropriate.

Three potential risk factors were identified from a thorough and well-focused literature review: restricted ankle dorsiflexion, obesity and time spent weightbearing.

In recognition of the importance of accurate measurement it is vital that these three factors were measured accurately. The study used a goniometer, which although a clinical technique that yields reasonably reliable results, may not truly reflect the exact amount of motion available. However, as there are few alternatives, this seems reasonable. Nonetheless, small differences would need to be

ignored due to the small, but perhaps important, measurement error associated with the technique.

Obesity was measured using the patients' self-reported values for height and weight. This may at first seem unreliable, but in support of this method the authors cite a study which suggests that patients' estimates are reasonably accurate.

Time spent weightbearing was assessed simply by asking the patient 'Do you spend the majority of your workday on your feet?' and 'Do you run or jog on a regular basis?' These questions could be viewed as reducing a complex issue to a simple yes/no answer and therefore must be regarded as a poor method of ascertaining this information. For example, how reliable do you consider public estimates of alcohol consumption or diet? Mmmmmm!

Case-control studies require clear definition of both groups. Cases were 50 consecutive patients with unilateral plantar fasciitis who presented at either of two designated clinics. Diagnostic criteria that mirror those used in other studies were used, strengthening the authors' assertion that their cases did truly have plantar fasciitis. Cases were selected from a local outpatients department – although the conditions they were presenting with were not recorded – and controls from a local church congregation. They were matched to the cases on the basis of age and gender, but did not have plantar fasciitis. These group definitions appear reasonable, although there does appear to be scope for more information.

Based on the foregoing, the method seems reasonable, but because of concerns over the precision of the measurement techniques, a large effect would have to be identified for the results to be believed. However, the examiner was not told whether each subject being assessed was a case or a control, and this blinding strengthens the method.

Overall, the methodology seems appropriate, although there are some concerns over the absolute accuracy of control recruitment and the measurement of the key study variables. Before reading the results we would be prepared to accept that this study has the potential to provide useful information on the role of ankle range of motion and obesity. However, the results concerning time spent weightbearing we would take with a 'pinch of salt' due to the weak method used to measure this variable.

CONCLUSION

Critical appraisal involves an analysis of a published research article and is performed to help us decide if the research is of sufficient quality to be used to inform our practice. We can perform a critique on various levels. We can begin by examining whether each section of the report provides the relevant information, using the IMRAD approach. We can then adopt a formal critical appraisal system which provides a series of questions relating to specific issues and results in a quality score. Appraisal systems range from the pragmatic and user-friendly Critical Appraisal Skills Programme (CASP) to the CONSORT statement which is used regularly to inform the design of appraisal tools by 'professional' researchers when conducting systematic reviews. All healthcare professionals who regularly read research papers – which should be them all – should familiarize themselves with both the CASP and CONSORT statement, and newer tools that have been developed in the same way as CASP. For example the MOOSE (Meta-analysis of Observational Studies in Epidemiology) and STROBE (Strengthening the Reporting of Observational Studies in Epidemiology) guidelines. The website addresses for CASP, CONSORT, MOOSE and STROBE are provided at the end of the book.

Expertise in critical appraisal will develop as we learn more about research design. Therefore, although we may not want to design a research study ourselves, our ability to read and evaluate research studies that could influence our practice will develop as we learn about research methods. Due to the inherent limitations of the peer-review process employed by the journals publishing research studies, we have a duty to learn more about the process so that we can make informed judgements on the quality of research and improve the evidence on which we base our practice.

REFERENCES

Black D 1998 The limitations of evidence. J R Coll Physicians Lond 32:23–26

Bland M 2000 An introduction to medical statistics, 3rd edn. Oxford University Press, Oxford

CASP 2006 Critical Appraisal Skills Program. Learning and development. Public Health Resource Unit, Milton Keynes Primary Care NHS Trust, Oxford. Online. Available: www.phru.nhs.uk/casp

Crombie IK 1996 The pocket guide to critical appraisal. BMJ Publishing, London

Gomm R, Needham G, Bullman A 2000 Evaluating research in health and social care. Sage, London

Gordis L 2004 Epidemiology, 3rd edn. WB Saunders, Philadelphia

Greenhalgh T 2000 How to read a paper: the basics of evidence based medicine, 2nd edn. BMJ Books, London

Greenhalgh T 2006 How to read a paper: the basics of evidence based medicine, 3rd edn. BMJ Books/Blackwell Publishing, Oxford

Hill A, Spittlehouse C 2001 What is critical appraisal? Bandolier Knowledge Zone. Online. Available: www.jr2.ox.ac.uk/bandolier/learnzone.html

Kannel WB 1990 CHD risk factors: a Framingham study update. Hosp Pract 25:119–127

Landorf K, Keenan A 2000 Efficacy of foot orthoses. What does the literature tell us? J Am Podiatr Med Assoc 90:149–169

MacAuley D, McCrum E, Brown C 1998 Randomised controlled trial of the READER method of critical appraisal in general practice. BMJ 316:1134–1137

Miettinen O 1998 Evidence in medicine: invited commentary. Can Med Assoc J 158:215–221

Moher D, Schulz KF, Altman DG 2001 The CONSORT statement: revised recommendations for improving the quality of reports of parallel-group randomized trials. J Am Podiatr Med Assoc 91:437–442

Moseley JB, O'Malley K, Peterson NJ et al 2002 A controlled trial of arthroscopic surgery for osteoarthritis of the knee. N Engl J Med 345:1719–1726

Oxford Centre for Evidence Based Medicine 2001 Online. Available: www.cebm.net

Polgar S, Thomas S 2000 Introduction to research in the health sciences, 4th edn. Churchill Livingstone, Edinburgh

Riddle DL, Pulisic M, Pidcoe P, Johnson RE 2003 Risk factors for plantar fasciitis: a matched case-control study. J Bone Joint Surg 85A:872–877

Rowan K 2001 The development and validation of a multi-dimensions measure of chronic foot pain: the ROwan Foot Pain Assessment Questionnaire (ROFPAQ). Foot Ankle Int 22:795–809

Tanenbaum S 1999 Evidence and expertise: the challenge of the outcomes movement to medical professionalism. Acad Med 74:757–763

Vetter NM, Matthews IP 1999 Epidemiology and public health medicine. Churchill Livingstone, Edinburgh

Chapter 6

The what and why of research

When you have eliminated the impossible, that which remains, however improbable, must be the truth.

Sir Arthur Conan Doyle

LEARNING OUTCOMES

By the end of this chapter you will be able to:
- Define 'research'
- Describe the key characteristics of the scientific method
- Discuss the major stages in research planning
- Discuss the major decisions involved in designing research
- Describe the process of hypothesis testing, and the factors influencing the choice of descriptive and inferential statistics.

Case Study

Why do we need to know about research methods?

In Chapter 5 a case study was presented concerning the critical appraisal of a research paper. This paper was titled 'Risk factors for plantar fasciitis: a matched case-control study'. Some key issues surrounding critical appraisal were highlighted and discussed, but several may still seem complex because we are not yet truly familiar with them. For example, whilst the concept of a case-control study may seem logical, when is this study design selected and what information can one provide? What do the terms *bias*, *chance* and *confounding* mean in reality? The definitions of these terms may be logical, but their relevance and application require further exploration to develop a pragmatic understanding. There is, therefore, a need to increase our familiarity with research and a variety of surrounding issues, generally.

This chapter will consider the nature, philosophy and key characteristics of modern research to provide greater insight and understanding. This increased knowledge and awareness will be invaluable in informing our appraisal and taking it to a higher, more detailed, level of understanding.

INTRODUCTION

Chapter 5 introduced the concept of critical appraisal together with information on specific questions that can be asked when evaluating the quality of published literature. Whilst brief explanations for, and justifications of, these questions were provided, it is likely that some uncertainty remains concerning, for example, terminology, the concepts involved or the relevance of specific issues. This chapter will complement Chapter 5 by exploring such issues in greater detail, beginning by defining, and considering the characteristics of the modern approach to, research. It will then proceed to consideration of research planning and implementation, and how the data gathered should be analysed. Whilst this information is clearly important when actually conducting research, an awareness of the issues involved also informs critical appraisal, helping us to develop as more informed, discerning and confident research consumers.

WHAT 'RESEARCH' IS, AND WHY WE DO IT

To begin with, we must develop a robust understanding of exactly what research is. A dictionary definition adequately conveys the spirit of the subject in terms of the discipline as applied to healthcare. For example, *Chambers Dictionary* (1998) defines it as 'a careful search…systematic investigation towards increasing the sum of knowledge'. This accurately reflects definitions that can be found in dedicated research texts. For example, Polgar and Thomas (2000) consider it 'a systematic and principled way of obtaining evidence for solving health care problems'. It can be concluded, therefore, that research is a *rigorous, controlled* and *ethical* approach to the collection of information to increase knowledge and understanding; these characteristics are integral to the discipline, as they increase the confidence we can place in the data gathered and conclusions drawn.

In broad terms, research is used to examine what we do as allied health professionals (AHPs) in an effort to ensure we are doing the best we can for our patients and also for society. 'What we do' encompasses a whole range of issues relating to clinical practice, including:

- the accuracy of diagnostic procedures
- the effectiveness of treatment regimes
- the techniques used for evaluating outcomes
- the adequacy of record keeping
- evaluation of health and safety issues within the clinical environment
- the effectiveness of infection control procedures.

Modern healthcare is complex, with AHPs utilizing a wide range of skills in their daily practice that includes, and extends beyond, these questions. The sphere of influence and importance of evidence-based practice has resulted in real pressure on all healthcare professions to demonstrate that their practice is clinically and economically effective and safe (Bristow & Dean 2003). Research, quite simply, is the key tool at our disposal to generate this evidence. To develop some idea of the enormity of the task now facing AHPs in developing the evidence required to support practice, it is useful to bear in mind that just 6% of AHP practice is considered to be underpinned by 'appropriate' evidence as opposed to 15% in nursing and 79% in medicine. These figures paint a sobering picture of AHP practice, in comparison to medicine especially, but it has been contended that favourable figures for medicine are flattering as the majority of medical research is, in fact, either too poorly done or insufficiently relevant to be clinically useful (Godlee 1998). Donaghy (1999) estimated that it will take 30 years before a suitable evidence base is established in the allied health professions. It is clear that for survival in a climate where practice underpinned by evidence is expected, ongoing programmes of quality research must be developed. 'Good quality' means research that has been well-designed, rigorously conducted and is clinically applicable. This chapter will consider some of the major issues influencing quality, but in the first instance the general philosophy and global characteristics of the process of research will be considered. These issues are conveyed in the *scientific method*, which developed during the *scientific revolution*, and their consideration provides a useful backdrop from which to go on to consider issues in research design.

KEY CONCEPT

The scientific revolution and the scientific method

Consider for a moment the questions 'How does our knowledge develop?' and 'How do we come to 'know' things?'

Clearly we do not simply accept as truth anything that anyone tells us. We have rules about what we will and will not accept as truth and we expect supporting evidence to be available. The scientific method describes the 'rules' used in contemporary science for deciding what evidence is required for information to be accepted.

The 'rules' have changed, however, throughout history. Those employed today are the result of an evolutionary process; this, quite correctly, implies that they will continue to evolve.

Understanding the *scientific revolution* and the *scientific method* fosters appreciation of the issues surrounding knowledge acquisition and verification, helping us separate fact from fiction to identify truth.

THE SCIENTIFIC REVOLUTION

The systematic, rigorous methodology that characterizes modern research is the result of much human endeavour, spanning many centuries and involving the work of numerous scientists and philosophers. Whilst scientists are busy conducting experiments to uncover 'truth', philosophers have considered how we ensure that the process of experimentation does, in reality, reveal truth. In effect, philosophers focus on the methods governing scientific endeavour in an effort to ensure that they yield trustworthy information. The scientific community has adopted a variety of approaches, each of which was felt logical and justified at the time, only to be later rejected as concerns were raised, deficiencies realized and solutions capable of providing more robust knowledge proposed.

The 'rules' governing contemporary scientific experimentation are encapsulated in *the scientific method*, which can be traced to *the scientific revolution*. This term is used to denote a series of events that occurred around 1600. Up until that time the theories and techniques developed by the Greek philosopher Aristotle (384–322 BC) underpinned knowledge acquisition. His approach involved the development of a theory followed by the gathering of supportive data. Modern research efforts, by contrast, operate on the premise that 'a few observations and much reasoning leads to error, many observations and a little reasoning to truth' (Carrel, cited in Talley & O'Connor 1996). Aristotle failed to appreciate this, although it is unfair to be too critical as his advances across many fields of study were impressive and undoubtedly laid foundations for those who followed.

Table 6.1 Important figures in the development of the scientific method

Figure	Dates	Contribution
Copernicus	1473–1543	Rejected the geocentric model of the universe, which placed Earth at the centre with the planets and sun revolving around it, in favour of the heliocentric system which placed the sun centrally. The idea seemed preposterous to most of his contemporaries and conflicted with religious belief that Earth was at the centre of the universe. This led to him being placed under house arrest.
Vesalius	1514–1564	Discredited Galen's views on physiology which included the four bodily humors: blood, phlegm, yellow bile and black bile. First proposed that the circulation of blood resulted from the beating heart and conducted some of the first human dissections, allowing him to assemble the first human skeletons.
Francis Bacon	1561–1626	Developed the philosophy of science, developing deductive reasoning proceeding from observation and experimentation. Although this model has since been developed, it represented a significant forward step. The rejection of any assumptions is a characteristic of modern science.
Descartes	1596–1650	Pioneered deductive reasoning. Sought to remove the influence of our biased thoughts from our observation in an effort to get back to pure truth.
Newton	1642–1727	Believed that scientific theory should be coupled with rigid experimentation.
Karl Popper	1902–1994	Refined the scientific method by asserting that theories can never be proved, only disproved, enforcing the concept that every theory should be systematically investigated to see if it can be overthrown. This premise is fundamental in modern research.

The concept that 'revolution' took place around 1600 is controversial (Shapin 1996), with some experts asserting that the sort of changes claimed to have taken place would, in fact, have occurred more slowly than the term 'revolution' implies (Kuhn 1996). Whether or not it is accurate to speak of a 'scientific revolution', key theoretical and experimental advances which influenced the methodology of scientific endeavour undoubtedly occurred around that time through the emergence of several philosophers who employed or developed a critical, unbiased approach which focused on systematic observation (Table 6.1). Key discoveries resulting from this new approach included those of Copernicus (1473–1543), who challenged the belief that the planets and sun revolved around Earth, and Vesalius (1514–1564), who performed the first human dissections, assembled the first skeleton and established that blood circulated because of the beating heart. Descriptions of the actual scientific method, and its key characteristics, were then presented by philosophers such as Sir Francis Bacon (1561–1626), who realized the value of observation and sought to gather as many as possible in the belief that truth would follow, and Descartes (1596–1650), who sought to remove the influence of our biased thoughts from observation in an effort to uncover truth. Bacon's description of the scientific method, however, was not fully accepted and further developments were required to produce the current method. This history provides strong reason to believe that further developments lie ahead. The work of Karl Popper (1902–1994), in particular, was seminal in the development of the scientific method as currently understood and practised.

EXERCISE

We are forced to the conclusion: that everything is the sum of the past and that nothing is comprehensible except through history.

Teilhard de Chardin (1959)

Using either an encyclopaedia or the Internet, review the contribution of the following individuals to the development of scientific methodology and progress:

Aristotle, Copernicus, Galileo, Bacon, Descartes, Newton, Einstein, Popper.

THE SCIENTIFIC METHOD

Whilst the Internet is a source of much misinformation, there are occasions when it is a rich source of knowledge. The scientific method, for example, is a topic well worth 'googling'. There have been numerous books and articles published on the topic, and many university departments have online teaching materials that provide good-quality accounts of the process. Table 6.2 shows the results obtained when the terms 'scientific revolution' and 'scientific method' were put into Google and Google Scholar.

As a case in point, the first hit returned when 'scientific method' was googled in December 2006 was *Introduction to the Scientific Method* from

Table 6.2 Internet searches concerning the scientific method: December 2006

	Google	Google Scholar
'Scientific method'	75 700 000	2 550 000
'Scientific revolution'	26 300 000	318 000

the University of Rochester in the USA (Wolfs 2006). This short, well-focused guide describes the scientific method as a four-step process:

1. Observation and description of a phenomenon or group of phenomena
2. Formulation of a hypothesis to explain the phenomena
3. Use of the hypothesis to predict the existence of other phenomena, or to predict quantitatively the results of new observations
4. Performance of experimental tests of the predictions by several independent experimenters and properly performed experiments.

The scientific method, therefore, is a process that begins with observation. This means that we measure what we see – it may be blood pressure, a health behaviour or a disease. The important aspect is that we utilize a valid and reliable instrument with which to record the observations so that we can have confidence in their accuracy. These observations are then used to formulate a hypothesis – a general statement explaining our observations. For example, going back to the case-control study example provided in Chapter 5, Alton Oschner, a 1940s surgeon, observed that many of his lung cancer patients smoked, which led him to hypothesize that there was a relationship between the two. The hypothesis is then used to predict new observations – for example, we might reasonably predict that there is a relationship between the amount of cigarettes smoked and the risk of lung cancer, or that stopping smoking will reduce the likelihood of developing the disease. The final step is absolutely key and is summed up in the phrase 'experiment is supreme'. This means that predictions should be examined through experimentation to provide information on the truth of the hypothesis. If we consider the development of knowledge concerning the effects of smoking, we can see that substantial evidence has accumulated over a long period of time to get to the current situation where it cannot realistically be contested that smoking has negative effects. In the scientific method experimental evidence is crucial, and a hypothesis cannot be accepted in the absence of such support.

A crucial concept in the scientific method is the paramount effort to remove the influence of our conscious thoughts to allow us to see clearly. We tend to find it difficult to remove the influence of, for example, upbringing, schooling, university education and other experiences, all of which influence our world view. The result is that these experiences can exert bias to affect, for example, the measurements we choose to record, the way we perform them, the individuals we select and our interpretation of the results. This concept can be traced back to Descartes' efforts to get back to 'pure truth' by minimizing as many sources of bias as possible to ensure that 'pure' observations are recorded. When we watch television detectives, such as Sherlock Holmes, Poirot or even 'CSI', it should strike us that a common thread is a quest for pure, unbiased facts gathered through observation, and clear identification of the facts. Watching these programmes after developing some knowledge of the scientific method will demonstrate the centrality of this theme.

One final principle underpinning the modern approach to research is the concept of scepticism – that anything can be challenged. This was introduced in Chapter 2 when it was stated by Pickering (1956) that: 'Half of what you are taught as medical students will in ten years have been shown to be wrong, and the trouble is, none of your teachers knows which half.' The truth of this statement is exemplified by history: consider that for all but some 250 years of our existence we believed that the world was flat. Black (1998) expressed this concept perfectly when he stated that: 'Every beautiful theory is vulnerable to an ugly fact…even a Newton awaits his Einstein.' It is interesting to consider which currently accepted truths will be shown to be inaccurate in the future (there will certainly be many examples), and this leads naturally to the concept that we should be sceptical of everything we do. However, this mustn't foster cynicism (believing that what we do doesn't matter because it's probably wrong anyway) – it is important that we strive to practise at the highest standard.

UNDERSTANDING HOW RESEARCH IS PERFORMED

Research should involve several clearly defined stages. Firstly, the approach should be planned, carefully considering the aim, and setting a hypothesis that is derived from a thorough literature review and is appropriately justified. An appropriate methodology must then be selected, on the basis that it will yield appropriate data related to the research question being investigated. Finally, the data must be analysed appropriately using techniques that are capable of revealing the information contained therein. To understand research and how it is performed, we must therefore consider issues surrounding research planning, research methodologies and data analysis, and the remainder of this chapter will be devoted to these issues.

RESEARCH PLANNING

The first step when conducting research is to thoroughly investigate the issue of interest, via a comprehensive literature review, to identify a gap in existing knowledge which needs to be filled. The information that is required to fill this gap must be expressed clearly. Firstly, this information requirement is expressed in terms of an aim, and from there it is refined into a hypothesis. For every study the data collected must be clearly related to the hypothesis – otherwise the information will be of little, if any, value in filling the knowledge gap identified. As the hypothesis drives both data collection and data analysis, and is the central foundation of every study, care must be taken when applying it.

FORMULATING A HYPOTHESIS

There are several steps that should be taken when developing a hypothesis and these are indicated in Figure 6.1. As can be noted, it is generally a process of increasing specificity.

For most steps identified the process is relatively straightforward: it is the derivation of a testable hypothesis that can be the most problematic, but this is also the most important. At this stage you have defined your research question in a broad statement and this needs to be broken down into smaller, more discrete units that can be studied. This is the hypothesis – a statement expressing the probable relationship between variables.

There are essentially two types of hypothesis: descriptive and directional. It is probable that you can tell the difference between the types just from their description. Descriptive hypotheses ask a specific question regarding some form of investigation. For example, what are the podiatric characteristics of those with lower back pain? A descriptive hypothesis, always framed in question format, would explore some aspect of the research question. For example, what is the distribution of foot type in those with lower back pain? Usually a descriptive hypothesis does not

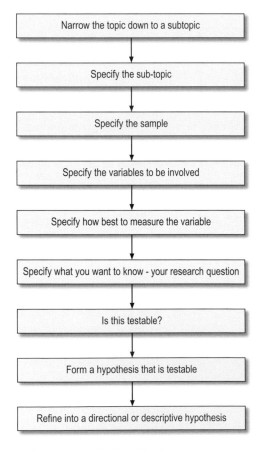

Figure 6.1 Process of developing the hypothesis.

include an active *independent variable*. If we do use an independent variable, then a directional hypothesis is required.

Directional hypotheses are phrased as a statement rather than a question. In these hypotheses the effect of an independent variable on a dependent variable is expressed. For example, in the statement, 'There is a relationship between foot type and lower back pain', the independent variable is foot type; the dependent variable, lower back pain.

Hypotheses need to be as specific as possible and deal with variables (e.g. behaviours, emotions, attitudes) that can be measured. If these variables are not clear or specific, the researcher should define the term. So, for example, if we are going to explore 'satisfaction' (e.g. if our hypothesis was 'Providing information leaflets will improve satisfaction in the podiatric clinic'), then we need to define and express how we are going to measure 'satisfaction'.

Suppose we are interested in the influence of environmental factors on practitioner performance in a podiatry clinic. We could express our research question as: 'What is the effect of environmental factors on practitioner performance in the podiatry clinic?' We would then have to define our terms and express how we are going to measure them (this process is known as *operationalizing* our terms). For example, environmental factors could be room temperature and noise. These could be operationally defined as:

- *Temperature* – amount of warmth in the air. Measured with a mercury thermometer using the Fahrenheit scale.
- *Noise* – amount of noise in the clinic as measured in decibels by a decibel meter.

In this study we can vary both the temperature and the noise and see how they affect practitioners' performance. Thus, temperature and noise are the *independent variables* and podiatric performance is the *dependent variable*. For several hypotheses (e.g. those relating to temperature) we may choose not to vary noise, but to hold it constant. In those cases when noise does not vary, it is a *control variable* instead of an independent variable.

Task

Write several hypotheses on the above study. Make sure that you operationally define 'podiatric performance'.

COLLECTING THE DATA

The experimental (scientific) method depends on physically measuring the variables as described in the hypothesis. The concept of measurement will be considered in detail later in this chapter, but for now it is important to introduce the concepts of numbers and units of measurement, of which there are several 'levels of measurement'. Each level corresponds to a different type of data, which is important because it determines how the data can be treated or analysed. Identifying the level of data is important since it not only provides direction for the researcher, but also allows the research consumer to have an overview of whether the analysis conducted in an article being read was appropriate.

THE NOMINAL LEVEL

These variables have a name value only (the word nominal means 'in name') and are the simplest of all. Examples of nominal level variables are sex (with the categories of male and female), religion (Catholic, Protestant, Jewish, Hindu, Buddhist, etc.) and foot type (pronated, neutral, supinated). The categories we form are simply the pigeon holes that we put people in to classify them. There is no order to them, neither implied nor intended, and inclusion in one category is either black or white (which is another nominal group!) – you either belong to a group or you do not. Since there is no order to these categories then we have to treat these variables as nominal and use appropriate statistical tests to examine the data.

THE ORDINAL LEVEL

The word ordinal means 'in order' and this provides an indication of the type of data that these variables assume. Ordinal data are those that have some order, for example social class where there is generally a top and a bottom. So, in our social class example we can classify individuals as Social Class I (upper class) through to Social Class V (working class). Another example would be the variable 'fear of scalpels' with categories such as very afraid, somewhat afraid and not afraid. A major use of ordinal level data is in those questionnaires that measure attitudes – for example, in Likert scales where categories may range from 'Strongly agree' through to 'Strongly disagree':

| Strongly agree | Agree | Neither agree nor disagree | Disagree | Strongly disagree |

These categories are in order and a rank is intended. However, the intervals between ranks are not assumed to be equal, thus the difference between the first and second rank is not necessarily the same as the difference between second and third.

As before, there is a range of statistical techniques that can be used with ordinal data and these are different from those used for nominal level data. By the same token, when ordinal data is assumed, powerful statistical techniques are not appropriate. Indeed, even the mean as a measure of central tendency (or average) should not be employed (the median is a more appropriate measure).

When collecting information for our study we could use nominal data; however, as this would restrict our statistical analysis we might wish to change it to ordinal. For example, when classifying patients visiting our podiatric clinic we could code according to reason: verruca, diabetes complications, plantar fasciitis and so on. This would be nominal data and restrict our analysis. We could change this classification so we classified them from least severe (e.g. verruca) through to most severe (diabetic foot) and therefore allow us to use different forms of analyses. However, this is obviously problematic and you have to ensure that your approach is sensible and valid.

THE INTERVAL LEVEL

Interval level data reflect some underlying dimension – just like with ordinal data – but with one crucial difference. Specifically, with interval measures numerically equal distances on the scale reflect equal differences in the underlying dimensions. The best, and most frequently used, example is temperature. Temperature is measured in degrees and not words (very cold, cold, OK, warm and hot) and these numbers correspond to the levels of mercury on a thermometer. The distance, or interval, between 11 and 12 degrees is exactly equal to the distance between 22 and 23 degrees, and between 68 and 69 degrees or 99 and 100 degrees. The intervals between any two adjacent categories are equal (exactly 1 degree).

THE RATIO LEVEL

Interval level data do not have a theoretical zero point – for example, temperature does not have a clear zero. There may be a zero on the thermometer but this does not indicate a lack or absence of temperature, it just means colder. Furthermore, there are different meanings of zero for one measure (i.e. Fahrenheit) compared to others (e.g. Celsius). For this reason, temperature is an interval level variable and not a ratio level variable.

The ratio level of measurement is the highest level since they have all the characteristics of the other levels but include a true zero point. An example is age – the categories have names (e.g. 5 years, 10 years, 22 years), the categories have an order from youngest to oldest, the intervals between the categories are equal, and it is possible to be zero years. Other examples include the number of children, years of education, years on the job, etc.

DESIGNING RESEARCH

After developing a research question and refining a hypothesis, the next challenge is to ensure that a good-quality study is designed: this means one that is capable of answering our question. Study design demands close attention to detail because if there are flaws then the results may be compromised. Petrie and Sabin (2005) state that poorly designed studies may give misleading results, and make the point that large amounts of data from a poor study will not compensate for design flaws. Therefore, it is important that we develop an understanding of the issues that determine study quality.

Research design is overwhelmingly driven by the concept of validity. In the broadest sense, validity refers to 'truth'. For example, if an 80-kg person stands on a set of scales which registers a value of 80 kg, then it can be claimed that they are valid, because they have measured accurately and truthfully. Whilst it is fairly simple to establish whether a set of scales is valid, the question 'Is this research study valid?' is more complex and does not have a yes/no answer: this is because it is dependent on not just one issue but on a whole range. For example, some important issues influencing the 'validity' of a research study include:

- the research design
- the sample studied
- the variables recorded
- the measurement techniques used for recording each variable selected

- the adequacy of the data analysis techniques used
- the appropriateness of the conclusions drawn.

Although numerous factors influence validity they need not be considered individually. This is because there are general categories which are useful for grouping issues. Inevitably there is some overlap between categories, with some factors having a legitimate claim to being included in more than one. Nonetheless, consideration of the major categories of validity represents a useful means of approaching the subject. These categories, which will be considered separately, are:

- measurement validity
- external validity
- internal validity.

MEASUREMENT VALIDITY

In relation to measurement, validity refers to whether a particular measurement instrument records the true value of the variable in question. For example, when a general practitioner measures blood pressure clinically it is important that the true value is recorded. The consequences of inaccurate measurement are twofold in that treatment may be provided when it is not actually required, or it may be withheld when it actually is required. Establishing the validity of clinical measurement of blood pressure can be definitively established through comparison of the clinical technique with those obtained using the gold standard – intra-arterial measurement. If the two techniques agree closely, then the clinical technique can be regarded as valid.

The assessment of blood pressure is, however, a relatively simple example; the assessment of validity is more complex in other situations. Consider pain. Pain can be assessed using a visual analogue scale where a 100 mm line is drawn with verbal anchors at each end (e.g. 'no pain at all' is written at one end and 'worst pain imaginable' at the other). The subject is asked to mark the point on the line which reflects their pain. The distance from zero is then measured using a ruler and taken as a measure of the pain the patient is experiencing. However, pain is a complex phenomenon which the visual analogue scale, whilst offering an insight to pain, undermines. By contrast, Rowan (2001) devised a foot pain assessment questionnaire which utilized a series of over 20 questions to provide more extensive information on the sensory (How severe is the pain?), cognitive (How does the pain make you feel?) and affective (How does the pain influence your behaviour?) aspects of pain. Whilst a visual analogue scale is a reasonable technique for rapid clinical assessment of pain, its limitations are clear.

Assessing the validity of an instrument can focus on one or more aspects, or dimensions, of validity. Prominent dimensions include *face, content, criterion* and *construct*. *Face* validity refers to the apparent suitability of the measurement tool on initial inspection: if it seems to fit the bill then it is, on the face of it, valid. Perhaps unsurprisingly this is regarded as weak evidence of validity (Gomm et al 2000). *Content* validity involves closer scrutiny to determine whether the separate dimensions of the variable are being measured: if it is known that there are a number of dimensions to a particular variable, and the instrument examines each one, the content is judged valid (Gomm et al 2000). Therefore, the Rowan foot pain assessment questionnaire, by considering sensory, cognitive and affective components of pain, achieves content validity. *Criterion* (comparative, predictive) validity involves the comparison of results obtained with the instrument under evaluation with those obtained using the gold standard technique (Daly & Bourke 2000). Finally, *construct* validity refers to the correlation between an instrument's score and clinically important outcomes such as prognosis (Gomm et al 2000). The key concept below offers a practical insight to the concept of validity. Whenever we use a measurement instrument, we must have an appreciation of its validity, otherwise we cannot claim to understand the results we obtain or their true significance.

KEY CONCEPT

Validity and *The Silence of the Lambs*

A study that utilizes a measurement instrument with questionable validity will yield questionable results – this represents a substantial threat to validity.

These concepts can be illustrated by considering *The Silence of the Lambs*. In one scene an FBI agent is sent to gather information from serial killer Hannibal Lecter in his prison cell. When passed a personality questionnaire, Lecter responds by stating: 'You think you can dissect me with this blunt little tool.' Clearly Lecter considered the questionnaire incapable of providing a valid insight to his personality! Devising a questionnaire that satisfies multiple validity dimensions for evaluating Lecter would be challenging, but to be valid the tool would have to do just that.

When considering which measure to use it is a useful idea to consider tools that already exist rather than use our own. For example, if we are interested in foot pain/function then there are various tools available that have been subjected to validation studies. These include the *Foot Health Status Questionnaire*, the *Foot Function Index* and the *Leeds Foot Function Inventory*. Bowling (2004) has produced an excellent text that reviews a multitude of tests that are available for measuring disease in various medical specialties, and is a useful source of quality information. The main advantages to using a prevalidated tool are that others will already have used it, giving it currency, and that extensive validation information should be available.

KEY CONCEPT

Measurement validity – the bottom line

All this information may make the issue of validity seem complex. However, remain focused by asking the same basic question of every measurement technique: 'Is it really measuring what it claims to be?'

EXTERNAL VALIDITY

When conducting a research study it is rarely, if ever, possible to include all the members of the population of interest. For example, a podiatrist who specializes in diabetes may be interested in the effects of a new type of footwear on the incidence of ulceration in neuroischaemic diabetics with a history of previous ulceration. Clearly it would not be possible – for economic, logistical and time reasons amongst others – to recruit all such neuroischaemic diabetics to the study as there are too many. A reasonable solution to this problem is to select a *representative* sample from the population and evaluate the intervention in this group. The ultimate aim would be to obtain results that could be applied to all neuroischaemic diabetics. This will only be possible if the sample recruited is truly representative of the wider population. The concept of sampling should not be new to us. For example, in *Masterchef*, judges do not eat all the food prepared by the aspiring chefs – they taste a sample of each dish on the assumption that this sample will provide an accurate insight to the quality of the food. Similarly, in *Pop Idol*, the judges are not forced (thankfully) to listen to a complete repertoire from each contestant: it is assumed that the short excerpt they do sing will be representative of their ability and will provide enough information for the judges to make an accurate decision.

Theoretically, if an appropriate sampling technique is used, a representative sample will be drawn and it will be legitimate to apply the results of the study to the wider population. However, if you have watched programmes like the ones mentioned you may have identified some concerns with sampling, and therefore can appreciate that sampling techniques, despite being theoretically robust, do have limitations. When considering the external validity of a research study we are charged with identifying and critiquing these limitations. The characteristics of the sample are, by definition, the source of sampling limitations. Therefore, we must think about the sample and ask what exactly they represent. For example, if we are studying Achilles tendinopathy, and we rely on patients' self-diagnosis of the condition, we will undoubtedly recruit a real mixed bag of patients who will have a potential myriad of disorders. Such a group would be *heterogeneous* – different. However, a *homogeneous* group – who are similar – is not necessarily the solution to this problem. If subjects with laboratory-diagnosed cystic

---

EXERCISE

Sampling

The concept of sampling is simple to grasp: we have all tasted some sort of food and based our judgement of that food on this limited exposure. Whilst we may be resolute in our judgement, this does not mean that sampling is flawless. Would it be reasonable to judge, for example, calamari on the basis of the frozen supermarket offering, or would the Michelin-starred restaurant be a better bet?!?

Think of an example of sampling – perhaps one of the examples above or one drawn from personal experience – and consider the ways in which it may be flawed.

What steps could be taken to minimize these potential flaws?

degeneration of the tendon only were recruited, then the findings may not be legitimately applied to subjects who have any other form of tendinous changes that could actually be considered within the spectrum of Achilles changes that denote tendinopathy! They are too narrow to be practically useful. The trick is to recruit a sample which falls somewhere in between, where we closely define our sample but ensure that the definition encompasses a practically useful 'cluster' of the condition.

Issues in sample selection

It is critical that when selecting a sample some important rules are followed. Firstly, an appropriate technique should be used to maximize the likelihood of recruiting a representative sample. Secondly, that sample should be large enough to maximize the likelihood of obtaining an accurate result. Both of these issues warrant further, separate, consideration.

Sample selection requires more thought than it may originally appear. It is simple enough if we have a series of individuals who are more or less the same – for example, if we are conducting a survey of student satisfaction amongst a group of students who all gained entry to university via A levels with a point range of 260–320, are all between 18 and 22, originate from the same geographical location and have the same ethnicity, then a random selection will suffice. However, as you are no doubt aware, it is highly unlikely that any researcher will obtain a distinct, well-defined group as this. It is more realistic that students will have gained entry through a variety of different qualification routes, will have a wide age range, a wide geographic origin and have a variety of ethnic origins. The sampling technique in this case would aim to ensure that students from each background category are represented. For example, if 40% of the students were between the ages of 18 and 24, 45% between 25 and 34, and 15% over 35, then the optimal sampling technique would recruit 40% of the sample from the 18–24 age group, 45% from the 25–34 age group, and 15% from those over 35. The sampling technique employed is determined by the nature of the population from which the sample is drawn. Many sampling techniques have been described, and the issue can be studied in detail. Some of the more common techniques were described by Kirkwood and Sterne (2003):

- *Simple random*: The required number of individuals is selected at random from the *sampling frame* – a list or database of all individuals in the population. The objective is for all individuals to have an equal chance of being selected.
- *Systematic*: For convenience, selection from the sampling frame is sometimes carried out systematically rather than randomly, by taking individuals at regular intervals down the list, with the starting point chosen at random. For example, if a 20% sample is required from a population of 100, this means that 20 individuals need to be selected. A number between 1 and 5 is randomly selected and then every fifth number is selected. For example, if 4 is the random number, then individuals 4, 9, 14, 19, 24, 29, 34 and so on are selected.
- *Stratified*: A stratified sample is taken when it is important to include distinct subgroups, so that all are adequately represented. A simple

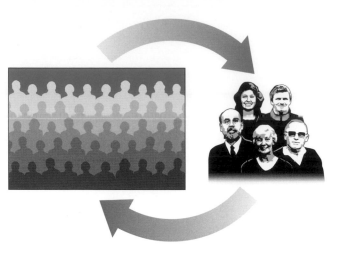

Figure 6.2 Sampling theory. If we select the sample carefully, then we may legitimately apply the results back to the population from which they were drawn.

random sample is then obtained from each distinct stratum. A proportional approach can be taken.

- *Multi-stage/cluster*: This type of sampling is carried out in stages using the hierarchical structure of a population. For example, a two-stage sample might consist of first taking a random sample of schools and then a random sample of children from each school.
- *Time-based*: For example, the 1970 British Cohort Study (BCS70) is an ongoing follow-up study of all individuals born between 5th and 11th April 1970 and still living in Britain.

If we get the sampling technique correct and they truly are representative of the population from which they were drawn, then it is legitimate to apply the study conclusions back to the sample (Fig. 6.2).

KEY CONCEPT

A representative sample

Sampling is concerned with selecting a group of subjects whose characteristics closely match or are identical to the wider population from which it is drawn. If the characteristics of the sample and the wider population match, then it can be said to be *representative*.

There are numerous techniques available for selecting a sample. However, it must be remembered that there remains a possibility that patients with certain characteristics may be over- or under-represented. As such, it is useful to evaluate if the sample does indeed match the characteristics of the original population.

Sample size

After identifying an appropriate sampling technique, it is then important to ensure that an appropriate number of subjects are recruited. This is important because whilst we want to ensure that important results are

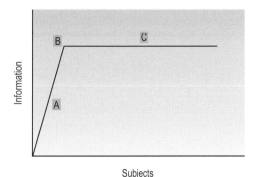

Figure 6.3 Illustrating the concept of sample size. As we recruit subjects we travel up diagonal line A, gathering new information. The apex of this line, B, represents the point where no more information is obtained. Too small a sample size will provide inadequate information as we do not reach point B, whilst recruiting a large sample size may take us far into the plateau, to point C. The aim is to get safely to the plateau without using up resources travelling too far into it. This would be represented by somewhere soon after B on the way to C.

not missed, we do not want to waste resources studying lots of subjects unnecessarily. In practical terms this can be thought of as information saturation: as we study any subject, a learning curve occurs as we recruit subjects, but this eventually flattens off. The optimal sample size takes us safely to the plateau (where we have gathered all the information we need) but does not lead us endlessly along it (Fig. 6.3).

The danger of recruiting an inadequate sample size is that we may make an error in the conclusions we draw. There are two errors it is possible to make, referred to as type I and type II errors:

- type I error – we reject the null hypothesis when it is true
- type II error – we do not reject the null hypothesis when it is false.

A study that recruits an appropriate sample size has, by definition, a low likelihood of incurring a type I or type II error and a high likelihood of detecting an effect if it exists. The sample size required for any particular study is determined by various factors:

- *The power required*: The power of a study refers to the chance of detecting an effect if it exists. A power level of $\geqslant 80\%$ is usually selected.
- *The significance level selected*: The significance level relates to the results of any statistical test we perform on the data. We decide at the design stage the numerical results returned by the test which will lead us to accept the null hypothesis. Statistical tests, and the concept of statistical significance, will be discussed further later in this chapter.
- *The variability of the observations*: To appreciate the significance of differences in a variable between two groups we need to have, in the first instance, information on the normal values for this variable in the population we are studying.

- *The smallest effect of interest*: We must be able to state the smallest effect considered important. For example, if we are evaluating the effect of a programme aimed at helping smokers cut down the number of cigarettes they smoke each day, we need to express the smallest reduction in the number of cigarettes that would be regarded as important. If a group smokes an average of 40 cigarettes a day, then a reduction of 10 cigarettes a day (equating to a 25% reduction) could perhaps be considered the smallest effect of interest.

Sample size is determined by the relationship between these four variables, and can be calculated using formulae, quick formulae, special tables, Altman's nomogram (a special diagram) or computer software (Petrie & Sabin 2005). Without exception, the sample size required increases as the:

- size of the effect of interest becomes smaller
- the significance level of interest increases
- the variability of the observations in the population increases
- the power level required increases.

In a published study it is common to see a power statement such as '75 subjects were required in each group for the *t* test to have an 85% chance of detecting a difference in means of 4 at the 5% significance level'. Such issues will be discussed further later in this chapter.

INTERNAL VALIDITY

Whilst external validity is a distinct, universally acknowledged concept, 'internal validity' is less so. This is because, although there is a general concept involved, it is common to see the term used in relation to 'causal' research or even omitted completely from texts providing detailed discussions of validity (e.g. Kline 2000, Murphy & Davidshoffer 2005). Coolican (2004) used the term to describe a situation where the results obtained in an experiment may have had nothing at all to do with what the researcher did. In such situations the study design has been internally flawed, and has failed to consider factors other than those of experimental interest, which may have exerted an influence. The term does, however, carry useful connotations when used beside the terms 'external' and 'measurement' validity. As such, in this situation it is defined as the adequacy or ability of the research design for providing truthful information relating to the research question.

For a study to have any hope of providing truthful information, or yielding accurate information in relation to the question it was designed to tackle, it must be free from bias and confounding. The illustration below provides an insight into how results can be influenced by participants. In a useful discussion of 'threats to internal validity', Coolican (2004) considered the influence that participants may wield, but also listed a variety of other mechanisms that may interfere with and corrupt any particular study to produce artificial results.

The factors presented Table 6.3 are not always discussed as 'threats to internal validity' and neither are they exhaustive. The terms *bias* and *confounding* are also in common use. It is, to all intents and purposes, appropriate to think of bias and confounding as describing threats to internal validity. For example, Gordis (2004) (who devoted a chapter of

Table 6.3 Threats to internal validity (after Coolican 2004)

Threat to internal validity*	Explanation of term
Using inappropriate statistical tests	May provide inaccurate results and therefore inaccurate conclusions
'Fishing' – 'shotgun' approach to data analysis by using lots of tests	Increases the likelihood of a 'chance' significant result occurring artificially
Reliability of measures and procedures	If the measurements or procedures used are not reliable, or if their reliability is unknown, it is impossible to determine accurately the implications of the effect
Random errors	Errors that occur simply by chance
Participant variation	In the example of group comparisons, it is important that participants in both groups have the same characteristics: if they are different, then these differences may account for the effect measured
History	Events which occur during a study which the researcher did not intend, or does not identify, could result in the effect observed
Maturation	Studies taking place over even modest time periods may see participants mature. A simple example is with child development studies
Testing	There can be a learning effect amongst participants, so that with repeated testing their knowledge of the test influences their performance, not their actual ability
Instrumentation	'Perfect' instruments do not exist. The error associated with any instrument being used needs to be understood for the results to have meaning
Selection bias	Selection bias can have many origins. For example, if an advertisement is used to identify potential subjects, keener, more motivated subjects may be over-represented
Drop-out	Particular types of subject may be more likely to drop out, and therefore the characteristics of the group change from that originally recruited
Imitation of treatment	If there is any contact between subjects from different study groups, there may be a change of behaviour, in either direction, based on perceptions about the treatment being received
Rivalry/demoralization	Some subjects may be motivated to 'do better' than other subjects

* Categories represent mechanisms through which various factors may act to bias or confound the results of an experiment.

his excellent – and highly recommended – textbook on epidemiology to these concepts) describes selection and information bias as mechanisms by which the validity of a study may be compromised. The routine use of these terms demands a robust definition. Gordis (2004) defined bias as 'any systematic error in the design, conduct or analysis of a study that results in a mistaken estimate of an exposure's effect on the risk of disease'. Confounding relates to the situation where a possible 'causal' relationship has been identified by a study. However, in this circumstance, the possibility that another factor could be responsible for the observed effect must be considered (Gordis 2004). Perhaps the simplest example of this relates to early research into the association between smoking and lung cancer. Several studies also identified that lung cancer seemed to be associated with alcohol intake. In this situation, alcohol intake was a confounding factor – obscuring or confusing the true relationship between smoking and lung cancer. In this situation the tendency for smokers to drink created the illusion that alcohol intake caused lung cancer when it did not.

It is difficult, time-consuming and unnecessary to discuss at length the numerous mechanisms by which bias and confounding may act. In any case, that would be missing the point: just as we are charged with examining the sample to determine if there is some unaccounted for characteristic that could be influencing the results, we are also charged with examining the method in an effort to identify potential sources of bias. Table 6.3 provides a guide to where bias and confounding may arise, and, by thinking about these in the context of each particular study we are appraising, we can begin to evaluate the particular ways in which that study may be compromised (Fig. 6.4).

EXERCISE

Select a study at random and read only the method. Setting aside the actions of the researcher, how many other possible explanations for any outcomes observed can you identify?

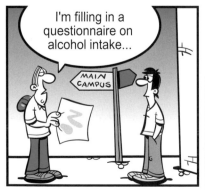 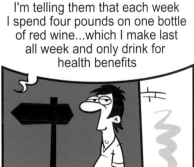 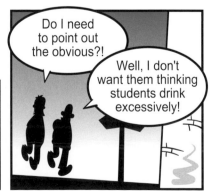

Figure 6.4 This cartoon superbly illustrates the problem of bias. It is not clear if the terms 'malicious' or 'humorous' bias exist, but perhaps they could be adopted to describe the provision of blatantly wrong information for personal amusement!

KEY CONCEPT

Bias and confounding

To develop an appreciation of biasing influences, consider the following:
'Clinicians encounter many patients taking prescribed medication, and a range of attitudes towards these drugs.'
Think of the reasons patients give for taking, or refusing to take, medication. Do you think that, in the context of a research study, such influences could act?

CHOOSING THE RIGHT KIND OF STUDY

After considering sample selection, the next step is to consider exactly what to do with it. This question relates to the type of study that is to be conducted. There are numerous different study designs available and each has its own unique characteristics. These characteristics determine the type of information obtained and what this information will mean. It follows that the choice of design is driven by the research question being asked. Knowledge of prominent research methodologies is vital for two reasons:

1. It helps researchers select an appropriate design that will yield information of value in answering their research question.
2. It helps clinicians (research consumers) determine whether an appropriate methodology was chosen for any study they are critically appraising.

This seems logical, but it is unfortunately inevitable that researchers may have to employ a method that is more convenient (or cheaper, or easier) than the design they really should have chosen. This frequently leads to the mistake of drawing inappropriate conclusions from the data obtained. One of the most common manifestations of this mistake occurs in relation to the randomized controlled trial. This methodology was designed to rigorously compare the effectiveness of more than one treatment for a condition. However, if a treatment makes a problem better, it is flawed to assume that the cause has been tackled. Greenhalgh (1996) called this pattern of reasoning the 'diagnosis by therapeutic response' approach. There are numerous situations where treatments make a patient better without tackling the cause: antibiotics decrease the pain and symptoms of an infected onychocryptosis...diclofenac sodium may make an Achilles tendinopathy feel less painful...a wax bath may make an arthritic foot transiently less painful. However, in each situation the effect is merely symptomatic, with the root cause remaining. For example, it is not until the offending nail is removed that the onychocryptosis can reasonably be expected to resolve. This clearly illustrates why randomized controlled trials should not be used to investigate cause: although the examples may appear simplistic, it has been convincingly argued that evaluation of

CLINICAL TIP

Remember the purpose and *pragmatic limits* of each research design. This ensures that appropriate inferences will be drawn from the data obtained.

Drawing conclusions that extend beyond the limits of the design employed is one of the most common errors made by researchers.

cause exceeds the theoretical and pragmatic limits of the RCT design (Miettinen 1998).

Although it may appear that there are many different types of research, there are, in fact, only a core cluster of research fields. These were introduced in Chapter 5 when their general characteristics were described. Greenhalgh (2006) described the broad fields of research as follows:

- *Therapy* – evaluating the effectiveness of treatments
- *Diagnosis* – evaluating the accuracy of diagnostic tests/procedures
- *Screening* – investigating the value of interventions aimed at detection of disease in the population
- *Prognosis* – investigating the impact of early detection of intervention on outcomes
- *Cause* – determining the role of particular agents on the development or progression of disease or illness
- *Psychometric* – evaluating attitudes or beliefs to help us understand how patients feel about the services or treatments provided to them.

Each field of research will be considered in turn to provide insight to its purpose, application and characteristics.

EVALUATING THERAPY

A question with clear implications for every practitioner on a day-to-day (if not hour-to-hour) basis is: 'What is the best way to treat this condition?' In modern healthcare we are faced with a situation where multiple treatments are available for most conditions. The challenge, therefore, is to select the best available intervention from those available. The randomized controlled trial (RCT) is considered the ideal design for evaluating the effectiveness and side effects of interventions (Gordis 2004, Greenhalgh 2006).

Various research books provide historical accounts of this design, providing interesting and useful insights. For example, in the foreword to Greenhalgh (2000), Weatherall recounts the story of Frederick II (1192–1250 AD), who was interested in the effects of exercise on digestion. After feeding two knights identical meals, one was allowed to sleep whilst the other was sent out hunting. After a few hours both were killed to determine how far digestion had progressed, and it was found that exercise inhibits digestion. Another equally brutal example, whilst never actually conducted, is worth repeating:

> In the 17th century Jan Baptista van Helmont…became sceptical of the practice of bloodletting. Hence he proposed what was almost certainly the first clinical trial involving large numbers, randomization and statistical analysis. This involved taking 200–500 poor people, dividing them into two groups by casting lots, and protecting one from phlebotomy while allowing the other to be treated with as much bloodletting as his colleagues thought appropriate. The number of funerals in each group would be used to assess the efficacy of bloodletting.…

In addition to providing insight to the RCT, this example also demonstrates the value of ethics!

Although numerous such historical examples of clinical trials are offered in the literature, Vetter and Matthews (1999) state that the concept of randomization can be traced to Fisher in 1935 and that the first clinical trial of recognized significance was performed for the Medical Research Council in 1946 by Austin Bradford-Hill. The trial concerned the effectiveness of streptomycin for tuberculosis and employed various design features that were directly intended to improve the quality of the trial. The concept of the RCT is elegantly simple: take a group of subjects, who are similar in important ways, and randomly allocate them to receive either treatment A or treatment B. Identify useful measures of success such as disease activity or symptoms, and record baseline measures prior to the commencement of the trial. Do not tell those providing, recording or receiving the treatments to which intervention they have been allocated, and repeat the measures after the treatment. These steps are taken to eliminate sources of bias, and by identifying which group fared better it is possible to state which treatment is better.

The RCT is characterized by its use of various design features that are felt to improve the quality of the results. These features include the following:

- Using well-defined diagnostic criteria, subjects eligible for treatment are identified.
- A suitable sampling technique is utilized, where possible stratifying according to important subgroup characteristics.
- Suitable 'control' and 'placebo' treatments are selected.
- Appropriate outcome measures are selected and are measured using a valid and reliable technique.
- A cross-over manoeuvre occurs to show that the strength of the response is linked to the treatment.
- Subjects and investigators are 'blinded', minimizing any bias that may arise from knowledge of who is receiving what treatment.

These characteristics are explicitly designed to reduce the elements of bias that may creep into the trial to distort results. Just as this design can identify positive benefits of treatment, it should be noted that it is also a very useful design for examining side effects. For example, if there is concern over any particular adverse effects, these can be selected as the outcome measures alongside any treatment benefits. A very much 'dumbed-down' version of the RCT is the 'Pepsi challenge' which formed the basis of a TV ad campaign in the late 1980s. Stalls were set up in public places and members of the public were invited to come and choose their favourite cola from two identical plastic cups which contained the same volume of liquid. Only after the participant had chosen would the cup be lifted up to reveal 'A' or 'B' to identify the cola chosen. This advertising gimmick demonstrates the advantages of randomization (the sampling order and subject selection), a control group (comparison of Pepsi with an alternative, control, cola) and blinding (the participant did not know which cola was being tasted), because any or all of these factors could have biased the results.

DIAGNOSIS

Accurate diagnosis is absolutely vital for effective clinical practice. History, physical examination and diagnostic tests combine to provide the required information to make an accurate diagnosis (Chou 2006), from which effective treatment and knowledge of prognosis follows. Inaccurate diagnosis may manifest in one of two ways:

1. a disease is diagnosed mistakenly
2. a disease is dismissed mistakenly.

Both possibilities have consequences. In the first situation a subject may be mistakenly subjected to treatment – which may involve the administration of toxic substances – or may be given worrying information concerning the course or prognosis of the disease mistakenly believed to be present. Whilst these possibilities are distressing enough, the consequences of the latter mistake are that vital treatment may be withheld. In many situations this will merely delay the instigation of treatment, but in other situations, where early treatment is vital to the prognosis, the inaccurate diagnosis may have fatal consequences (Gordis 2004). It is vital, therefore, that we understand the accuracy of the diagnostic procedures that we use in clinic.

Studies of diagnostic tests aim to determine their ability to detect the disease accurately if it is present and to reject the possibility of disease accurately where it is absent. A useful way of thinking about this concept is to consider how effective any particular test will be at separating out subjects with a disease from those without (Gordis 2004). A prerequisite for determining this information is knowledge of actual disease state, which is often determined using a 'gold standard' technique. Diagnostic studies involve completing a 2×2 table from which the sensitivity and specificity of a test can be calculated (Table 6.4). Sensitivity refers to the *ability to identify correctly those with the disease* whilst specificity refers to the *ability to identify correctly those without the disease.* This is sometimes remembered using the acronyms SnNout and SpPin (Chou 2006):

- *SnNout* – if sensitivity is high, a negative result rules out the disease
- *SpPin* – if specificity is high, a positive diagnosis rules in the disease.

This can be put into context by considering the example shown in Table 6.5, where figures are put into the cells in the table.

Realizing that few tests are 100% accurate leads clearly to the conclusion that the concepts of sensitivity and specificity must be understood for the effective use of diagnostic tests. Consider plantar digital neuritis (Morton's neuroma). Clinical investigation of this pathology includes mediolateral compression of the metatarsal heads combined with translation in a superior–inferior direction, with a 'click' or 'pop' felt or heard when a neuroma is present (Hyman et al 2006). To use this test most effectively it would be useful to have some idea of its sensitivity and specificity – this tells the clinician what weight to lend to the results. If the rates are high this brings confidence in the diagnosis, but if they are low then it indicates that other pathologies in the differential diagnosis should not be ruled out. Excellent discussions of these concepts were provided by Vetter and Mathews (1999) and by Gordis (2004), who also provided a worked example of how to evaluate the sensitivity and specificity of combinations of tests, reflecting the real-life clinical situation where multiple tests are often conducted simultaneously.

Table 6.4 Calculating sensitivity and specificity

Test result	Disease	No disease
	True disease status in population	
Positive	True positives (TP) (Have the disease and a positive test)	False positives (FP) (Do not have the disease but have a positive test)
Negative	False negatives (FN) (Have the disease but have a negative test)	True negatives (TN) (Do not have the disease and have a negative test)

Sensitivity = TP/TP + FN; Specificity = TN/TN + FP.

Table 6.5 Calculating sensitivity and specificity: a worked example*

Test	Disease actually present	Disease actually absent	Total
Test positive	8	10	18
Test negative	2	80	82
Total	10	90	100

* Figures refer to a population of 100 where 10 have the disease and 90 do not.
Sensitivity = 8/10 = 80%; specificity = 80/90 = 89%

EXERCISE

Sensitivity and specificity in clinic

List the five clinical tests you use most often – 'Mulder's click' is an example of one.

How robust do you consider each test to be? Can you justify your view? Is published information available regarding sensitivity and specificity for any of these tests?

KEY CONCEPT

Interpreting test results

A positive or negative test simply *suggests* the presence or absence of a particular disease. Few tests are perfect, and we must always remember that the test result may be wrong.

This concept refers equally to clinical, imaging and laboratory tests.

SCREENING STUDIES

Screening for disease involves the use of diagnostic tests to determine the presence or absence of the disease in question. Therefore, the concepts underpinning the evaluation of diagnostic tests apply here also. However, when a test is being used for screening purposes it is aiming to detect a disease early so that treatment can be provided. For screening tests to be effective it is vital that the process is cost-effective and that treatment is available. An ideal screening programme would:

- employ a test or procedure that has high rates of sensitivity and specificity
- be cost-effective, meaning that a test is cheap and frequently identifies patients with the disease
- result in effective treatment, thereby avoiding the prolonged/expensive/more invasive/more serious treatment associated with later diagnosis.

Public health medicine is concerned with achieving the greatest health benefit for the most people for the available money. In this respect it can be seen that it would not be the most effective use of resources to spend a lot of money performing an expensive, perhaps painful, test on a large group of people in the hope of identifying one person with a disease, especially if that diagnosis will not necessarily result in more effective treatment. The interpretation of data relating to screening programmes should deal with these issues so that the cost/benefit ratio can be evaluated.

PROGNOSTIC STUDIES

The prognosis of any particular pathology relates to the course it is likely to take and the eventual outcome. Information related to prognosis is important for a variety of reasons (Gordis 2004):

- It is necessary to understand the implications of treating that disease in order to establish priorities for clinical services and public health programmes.
- Patients often ask questions about the course they can expect their pathology to take and what the eventual outcome is likely to be.
- Prognosis is likely to change as new treatments become available, but the influence of new treatments can only be evaluated by comparison against the previous natural history of the disease.

Each pathology we see has its own unique natural history. A useful schematic representation of the natural history of a disease was presented by Giles (1997) (Fig. 6.5). This demonstrates how each pathology

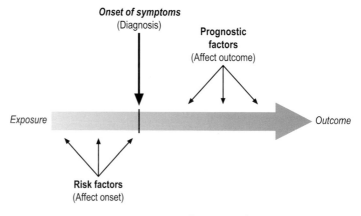

Figure 6.5 The natural history of a disease (Giles 1997).

begins to develop in response to a particular 'exposure': this could be some form of stimulus or basic biological event or defect. At this stage the symptoms are not present, but various other factors (e.g. lifestyle or activities) may influence the rate of progression, until symptoms are noticed, advice is sought and the diagnosis is made. After the diagnosis is made the disease will continue to progress towards the final outcome, although lifestyle modifications and medical interventions may be introduced to influence this outcome.

In order to provide patients with information on prognosis we must understand the natural history of the disease, preferably both with and without interventions. The preferred study design for investigating prognosis is the longitudinal study (Greenhalgh 2006), which involves taking a group of subjects and following them over a period of time to see what happens to them. Textbook discussions of prognostic studies focus on the 'big' diseases (e.g. cancer and heart disease) where the endpoint is death, and seek to explore the ways in which the time to death can be extended. Concepts such as the *case-fatality rate*, which refers to the number of people who die from the disease divided by the people who have the disease, and *person-years*, which describes the number of deaths divided by the person-years over which the group is observed. Whilst such data are relevant in certain specialties, such as the diabetic foot, it is clearly inappropriate to discuss the prognosis of a majority of podiatric pathologies using such terms. However, it is equally apparent that for the provision of accurate information to patients relating to the diagnosis of their pathologies, information relating to prognosis is vital. In these situations it is more appropriate to record serial measurements of disease status using meaningful tools. For example, to investigate the prognosis of plantar fasciitis, it would be appropriate to take serial measurements using the Foot Health Status Questionnaire (Bennett et al 1998). It would be important to ensure that an adequate follow-up time was allowed so that the true course of the disease is understood and not just a short-term snapshot.

Longitudinal studies involve the recruitment of subjects with a disease and following them over a period of time to determine how their pathology progresses. A necessary characteristic of such studies is that they are prospective, in that they recruit subjects and follow them up over a period of time. Factors that need careful consideration include the diagnostic criteria and the severity of the presenting symptoms. This is because weak diagnostic criteria and high variability in the presenting symptoms suggest considerable variation in disease severity which will confound the information obtained.

CAUSAL RESEARCH

'Causal' research is concerned with evaluating whether a putative harmful agent is related to the development of illness. This area of research is the domain of epidemiology, which can be defined as 'the study of the incidence, distribution and determinants of disease' (Wald 1996). This may seem a secondary priority, however, as it is not always necessary to understand the cause of a disease to treat it successfully: the clinician's traditional role has, after all, been with the treatment of established disease. On the other hand, there are several reasons that causal research is vital:

- It opens up opportunities for prevention. Opportunities for prevention demand knowledge of the factors either causing or influencing the progression of a disease in order that they can be influenced.
- Cause is inherently related to risk, and patients frequently want information on what they can do to reduce their risk or improve their symptoms, again necessitating information regarding causal factors.
- Clinical encounters often lead practitioners to develop a hunch regarding the cause of a particular condition and, as such, it is useful to understand how these hunches can be rigorously investigated.

Whilst 'cause' is relatively straightforward in the case of infectious disease, where, for example, the only way to develop AIDS is to be exposed to the human immunodeficiency virus, Gordis (2004) explained that modern disease tends to be chronic in nature and influenced by many factors. As such it becomes impossible to speak of a single cause: to apply this concept in these situations we need to consider the concepts of *necessary* and *sufficient* cause to explain the precise role of a range of factors involved in any particular disease process. For example, plantar fasciitis may be related to foot function, obesity, occupation or posterior muscle flexibility. However, whilst each factor may be a *sufficient* cause, in that it may produce the pathology independently of the other factors, it is not *necessary* – it is possible to develop the disease without being exposed to it.

The complexity of the relationship is compounded by the interaction of factors. Causal research, in modern healthcare, is complex and it can be difficult to isolate the role of individual factors. Concepts such as the *odds ratio* (which equates with betting odds and is usefully explained by Bandolier) can be calculated using information from case-control and cohort studies, and provides a useful method of expressing the increased risk of developing a disease associated with single and multiple exposures.

The major designs used in causal research are *cohort* and *case control*. Both these designs involve analysis of rates of disease in exposed versus non-exposed subjects, thereby permitting calculation of the rates of occurrence in the two populations. This demands that the rate of occurrence of the disease is measured, and the terms *incidence* and *prevalence*

Table 6.6 Expressing the risk of a disease associated with particular factors (Farmer et al 1996)

Measure	Description
Absolute risk	The most basic measure of risk: the incidence of a disease in any defined population
Relative risk	The ratio of the incidence rate in the exposed group to the incidence rate in the non-exposed group; sometimes expressed as a percentage
Attributable risk	The difference between the rate in the exposed and non-exposed groups; it represents the risk attributable to the factor being investigated

are commonly used for this purpose: incidence refers to the number of new cases in a defined time period; prevalence relates to the number of cases of the disease in a particular area at a particular point in time. These rates can then be manipulated in various ways to calculate a range of statistics (Table 6.6). However, establishing that a particular variable is associated with a particular disease demands that a series of criteria are fulfilled. These criteria are termed the 'criteria for inferring causality' and are discussed by most epidemiology textbooks (Box 6.1).

Box 6.1 The criteria for inferring causality (Wald 1996)

Essential criteria
- A real association, i.e. one that is unlikely to be due to chance
- Exposure to the factor precedes the onset of the disease
- The association cannot be reasonably explained by bias, either through systematic measurement error or through the effect of one or more confounding factors
- The causal explanation is biologically plausible

Additional criteria
- Strength of association: a relative risk as high as three or four times is less likely to be due to bias than one or two or less
- Consistency in the evidence from several studies that are unlikely to share the same bias
- Demonstration of a dose–response relationship between factor and disease
- The distribution and frequency of the disease in different groups and over time follows the distribution and exposure of the factor
- Support from in vivo or animal evidence

Although these criteria focus on information gained from cohort and case-control studies, it is worth focusing for a moment on some of the other criteria that are presented. For example, it makes sense that exposure to the factor should precede the development of the disease, and whilst this may seem so obvious that it does not warrant mention, there are situations when we take for granted a particular temporal relationship. As an example, consider a prominent study concerning the relationship between pronated feet and juvenile hallux valgus (Kilmartin 1994). Whilst it is widely perceived that pronation leads to hallux valgus (HAV), by the time Kilmartin had completed his study he began to seriously question the nature of the relationship (personal communication 2007), i.e. he began to entertain the possibility that whilst HAV and the pronated foot are related, the temporal relationship should not be taken for granted. Just because we see two features together does not necessarily mean that one caused the other: both may be caused by a third variable.

This leads on to consideration of another criterion – the biological plausibility of the causal explanation. Information should be sought in relation to the mechanism of action, or mode of influence, of the causative factor. For example, there is a 'believable' theoretical pathway by which pronation may result in hallux valgus, and this does lend weight to the possibility of a causal relationship acting in a particular direction. We should always look for this type of information, and laboratory studies – involving, for example, live patients, cadaveric specimens or mathematical modelling – can be very useful in establishing the precise pathway by which a factor results in the development of a disease. To illustrate this, consider the causal pathway by which cigarette smoke 'causes' atherosclerosis – the arterial pathology that can result in myocardial infarct, stroke or peripheral vascular disease. Clearly, for this agent to be accepted as a 'cause' of this disease, the exact mechanism of action had to be identified. In this way it can be seen that information from numerous sources is vital for a particular factor to be classed as a 'cause' of a particular disease.

PSYCHOMETRIC RESEARCH

The broad fields of research considered so far have concerned, for example, measurement of the presence or absence of a disease, the relationship between variables and the accuracy of a diagnostic test. Such research designs do not, however, consider how patients feel about the treatment they have received, the way they have been treated or the impact of a disease or treatment on psychosocial function. Such issues can only be evaluated by measuring attitudes, perceptions or beliefs, and this is normally done using some form of questioning. Questionnaires are usually made up of a number of *items* (questions or statements) which can be organized into several domains or dimensions, depending on the basis of your questionnaire. A domain or dimension refers to an area of functioning, experience, ability or some other characteristic that is being evaluated. For example, the Foot Health Status Questionnaire asks questions relating to several 'domains' contributing to overall foot health, including 'foot pain' and 'foot function'. If questionnaires have already been developed to measure the variable of interest, it may be possible to develop a questionnaire pack or 'battery of tests' based on a compilation from these questionnaires. This is, of course, relatively easy (although careful steps have to be taken in order to ensure validity and reliability of these composite measures). However, in other situations it may be that we are trying to measure a variable that has not been measured previously, and therefore it will not be possible to obtain an existing measurement tool. In such situations the questions to be put into the questionnaire must be developed.

Item generation

There are two approaches to developing questionnaires (for a fuller discussion see Upton & Upton 2007) – one could be called the clinical approach (or 'clinimetric approach') whilst the other could be considered more statistical (or the 'psychometric approach'). The first approach uses the opinions of patients and clinicians with the aim of developing measures that have face validity which make 'clinical common sense' (Feinstein 1999). Thus this approach is concerned less with the homogeneity of scale items (items that fit well together due to similarity) and more with their clinical relevance to a phenomenon. It is not uncommon, therefore, to develop a scale which includes heterogeneous items (items concerning a range of issues not immediately related, but all of which are useful). An example of the clinimetric approach would be to ask a group of patients or practitioners about the aspects they considered important in relation to a particular issue and generate questions from these.

In contrast, psychometric strategies (e.g. Marx et al 1999) rely more on statistical techniques and generally aim to develop a measure that is mathematically valid and reliable, which usually means a degree of homogeneity is valued. However, there is little difference between the two methods as quoted in the literature since 'each has its own merits... sometimes the best approach is to use both methods' (Feinstein 1999).

Furthermore, despite the claimed difference in aims and strategy, in practice there is some overlap between the two techniques and it is easy to see how they might be complementary. Indeed, Streiner (2003) goes one step further, cogently arguing that clinimetrics is a misnomer – the strategies referred to as clinimetric practices are simply a subset of psychometry.

So how can the items for the questionnaires be generated? The initial step is to generate as many items as possible – create the item pool. The derivation of an initial item pool is based on a combination of literature review and focus groups or interviews with the target population, and relevant professionals. It is not simply about the researcher sitting down and developing the items, although this forms a part – a range of systematic approaches is required. The literature review should always be your first port of call and you should always be systematic in your approach to the review (see Chapter 3). For example, when exploring teachers' effectiveness, Wotruba and Wright (1975) reviewed the literature and found 21 specific studies which they used as the foundation for their item pool, and subsequent interviews with teachers and relevant individuals (e.g. students) were used to expand this item pool.

Another method of obtaining items is through the use of focus groups. Focus groups involve the 'explicit use of group interaction to produce data and insights that would be less accessible without the interaction found in a group' (Morgan 1988, p. 12). The dynamics of the focus groups can foster the generation of numerous critical items which otherwise might not come about.

Focus groups can be seen as better than more traditional methods if there is no previous literature on the topic or you are uncertain over the type of information you require. Furthermore, the items can be modified in order to attain more appropriate terminology and wider appeal. Focus groups can be charged with this task, along with that of generating additional items.

On the other hand, individual interviews with professionals, patients or children can be held. For example, during the initial developmental stage of constructing a measure exploring attitudes towards health in children in local authority care, it would be important to carry out interviews (or focus groups) with children in care, foster carers, community paediatricians, health visitors and other relevant professionals such as social workers.

The divergence in methods lies in deciding which items to keep once this initial item pool has been developed. The clinimetric strategy relies on the ratings of patients and clinicians to determine which items to include in the final scale. Typically, patients may be asked to rate the importance of each of the items in the initial pool on a five-point scale from 'not at all important' to 'extremely important' so that a mean importance score can be determined for each item. The items with the highest scores will then be selected for the scale. Item selection using the psychometric approach usually relies on factor analysis, a statistical method which organizes items into factors according to their relationships with one another. Items selected for each scale therefore tend to have good homogeneity. Selection of items has been found to differ for the two methods, even when starting with the same item pool (Marx et al 1999), i.e. the items patients perceive as important are not necessarily the same as those which show statistical importance. However, it should be noted that it is not uncommon for a scale to be modified by a clinician in order to improve content validity, whichever initial method of item selection has been used (Marx et al 1999). Furthermore, it is also possible to combine both patient and statistical judgements in the choice of final items. The combined use of statistical analysis and human intuition is, according to Streiner (2003), a common combination in psychometrics.

Finally, the methods used to confirm the reliability and validity of the newly minted measure are the same for both psychometrically and clinimetrically derived measures. For Streiner, 'The conclusion is that clinimetrics is not describing a new family of techniques that should be used with a unique type of scale, but is simply another word for a portion of what is done in psychometrics' (Streiner 2003, p. 1144). Even ardent supporters of clinimetrics as a distinct method of questionnaire development accept that there is much overlap with psychometrics. Indeed, the distinction between the terms psychometrics and clinimetrics is often hazy as both disciplines at times make use of the same methodological and statistical approaches (de Vet et al 2003). The main difference, it seems, is in the emphasis given to patient and clinical opinion during item selection – in all other ways the practices of clinimetricians and psychometricians can be viewed as interchangeable.

HYPOTHESIS TESTING AND DATA ANALYSIS

Having decided on the method of generating data we can then go ahead and gather our data. This is the part of research that is perhaps perceived to be the main part – the actual 'doing it' bit. The reality, however, is that this is a small part of a much more involved process: devising an appropriate approach, as we have seen, requires much time, thought and effort that may dwarf the effort associated with data collection, and, similarly, we must carefully consider how we process the information collected to ensure that we fully understand its meaning. The purpose of the data analysis is to present some information, to compare the data or to explore relationships between the data. Whenever we approach this task it is useful to consider it explicitly in the context of *hypothesis testing*, i.e. we must remember that the data were gathered for the purpose of shedding light on the hypothesis that we took care to set. As such, we must think of our data analysis as the gathering and presentation of evidence related to the hypothesis that will help us draw a conclusion regarding whether we should accept or reject it. We must appreciate that statistics are simply tools that give us insight to the data we have collected, allowing us to form a conclusion on our hypothesis.

The first thing we need to do when we have collected the data is to describe them. To do this, two questions are initially useful: 'What is the average score?' and 'How many people sit in or around this value?' There are a number of methods of measuring the average (or measures of *central tendency* as they are known) and dispersion (the measure of *spread* of a variable around the average).

DESCRIPTIVE STATISTICS

Descriptive statistics do what they say on the tin – they describe the data in our study. They provide simple (but not simplistic) summaries of the sample and the measures, and should be in virtually every quantitative study. They are basically used to describe what's going on with the data and should present the data in a manageable form. Descriptive statistics help us to simplify large amounts of data in a sensible way. An excellent example of descriptive statistics in everyday life is the football league table, which synthesizes the results (and other performance indicators) of lots of matches in a straightforward and easy-to-access manner. The alternative to this would be to list the results of all the individual matches played and try to make sense of them. In the context of a podiatry study, suppose we had some 100 patients where Foot Posture Index had been measured. Presenting all these data in a table would be time-consuming, difficult to read and difficult to interpret. What we want is a simple measure of the average that would help us describe the data – this is what measures of central tendency provide. However, this does not tell us about the distribution around the central measurement. Therefore, it is useful to have a measure of this deviation from the average, and this is what the measure of variation will tell us.

Measures of central tendency

There are three major types of central tendency: mean, median and mode.

The *mean* is probably the most commonly used method of describing central tendency. To compute the mean all you do is add up all the values and divide by the number of values; this is what most people would describe as the average. The mean should only be used with interval and ratio data.

The *median* is the score found at the exact middle of the set of values. One way to compute the median is to list all scores in numerical order, and then locate the score in the centre of the sample. This should be used with ordinal data.

The *mode* is the most frequently occurring value in the set of scores. To determine the mode, you might again order the scores as shown above, and then count each one. The most frequently occurring value is the mode. This should be used with nominal data.

Dispersion

Associated with measures of central tendency are measures of dispersion and there are two main forms: the range and standard deviation. The range is merely the highest value minus the lowest value. Obviously one problem with this is that outliers at either end can exaggerate the range.

In contrast to the range, the standard deviation is a more detailed estimate of dispersion and shows the relation of the set of scores to the mean of the sample. The standard deviation is 'the square root of the sum of the squared deviations from the mean divided by the number of scores minus one'. Although this appears a rather complex formula, it can be calculated simply and many programs are available to help you with the maths (e.g. Excel or various web pages on the Internet).

EXERCISE

Statistics and hypothesis testing

Suppose you are interested in understanding the relationship between glycaemic control and pedal complication rate in non-insulin dependent diabetics. 250 consecutive non-insulin dependent diabetics, who have a disease duration of >5 years, are recruited from a diabetes clinic to examine the hypothesis: 'Glycaemic control influences pedal complication rate in NIDDM.'

Subjects are sorted, according to their average glycaemic control over the past 5 years, into one of three groups: good control, average control or poor control. In such a study the independent variable is glycaemic control and the dependent variable is pedal complications.

Write down some ideas concerning how you would organize a database and the descriptive statistics you could use to begin to gather evidence allowing a conclusion to be drawn.

Using the flowchart in Figure 6.7, determine the appropriate inferential techniques.

PARAMETRIC OR NON–PARAMETRIC

There are two forms of inferential statistical tests: parametric and non-parametric. Parametric tests are the more powerful type of tests and should be used whenever possible. However, they are based on highly restrictive assumptions about the type of data:

1. It is assumed that the data are drawn from a normal population. Although not a perfect method, one way of testing this is to simply draw out the data, which should result in a normal curve (Fig. 6.6). Although the normal curve highlights that most people are in the 'average' range (i.e. the shaded part of the graph indicated by a '0'), there are some in the extremes, and as we get further towards the extreme then there are fewer people in these groups. For example, if we took 1000 men and measured their height we would find that most would be average – 5 ft 11 in. However, we would have some men who were shorter, 5 ft (lighter blue on left), and a few who were even shorter, 4 ft (shaded white on left). Similarly, at the other end of the spectrum we would have some that were above average, 6 ft 3 in (lighter blue on right), and a few who were even taller, 7 ft (shaded white on right). An example closer to home relates to exam results: in the authors' 30 years teaching experience, there has never been an exam which yielded results which were not normally distributed!

2. The populations are assumed to have the same variance. Again, this is difficult to determine but can be simply examined by inspecting the 'spread' of the data. In Figure 6.6, how does the curve spread

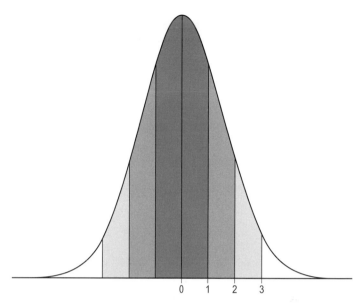

Figure 6.6 Normal peak.

away from the average? Is this similar to the other group you are comparing?

3. The variables are assumed to have been measured on the interval scale. We have discussed the assumptions that underlie an interval scale and these must be met for parametric tests to be used.

If these three conditions are met, then parametric tests should be used. On the other hand, if these conditions are not met, then non-parametric tests have to be used.

INFERENTIAL STATISTICS

Once you have described the data using your descriptive statistics then you can move on to the inferential statistics which allow you to draw conclusions that extend beyond simple description. For example, we may use statistics to compare the different groups, explore relationships between variables or infer from the sample what the population might be like.

Inferential statistical tests are techniques for helping us decide what the data we have gathered are telling us. For example, if we want to know if there is a relationship between foot type and lower back pain then we may measure the distribution of foot types in populations of subjects with and without lower back pain. If there is a connection between the two then we would expect the distribution of foot types in the two groups to differ. After gathering our data we could, using descriptive statistics such as mean and standard deviation, describe the foot types found in the two groups and this may suggest similarities or differences between the two. However, a more powerful way to look at this problem is to use an inferential test to ask the question: 'What is the probability that the sets of scores obtained from these two separate groups came from the same population?' The more similar the scores, the more likely the inferential test is

CLINICAL TIP

Statistical significance is all very well, but it is important to think in terms of *clinical significance*. The two do not always equate. If a statistical test result is telling you that two sets of scores are different, look at the average difference and the standard deviation. If there is a small difference between the two that you consider to represent an unimportant clinical effect, then think carefully before rejecting this clinical interpretation.

to conclude that these could have come from the same population and not two different ones. Inferential statistical tests calculate a '*p*' value, which in this example would relate to the *probability* that the two sets of scores came from two different groups: if there is a large difference in mean and standard deviation, for example, this would suggest that the two groups differ. However, if there is a small difference in the means with a similar standard deviation, then this could be satisfactorily explained by the normal variation that could be expected in a single population. The larger the difference, the more likely the groups are to be different. By convention, a *p* value of <0.05 is taken as indicating statistical significance, and is reported as a statistically significant result. This means that there is less than a 5% chance that the difference in the scores obtained between the two groups could have occurred by chance.

There are a myriad of statistical tests and the choice can be bewildering and confusing. However, rather than learn about each individual test, it is useful to begin by considering the decisions involved in selecting a test. If we understand these factors then we can negotiate the flowcharts provided in textbooks that show which test should be used in which situation. These can get quite complex, but at the most basic level the choice of test is determined by the level of data and the number of groups being compared. For example, if you want to compare the average between two groups when you have collected interval data you should use a *t* test for differences between groups (Fig. 6.7). If you wanted to look at the

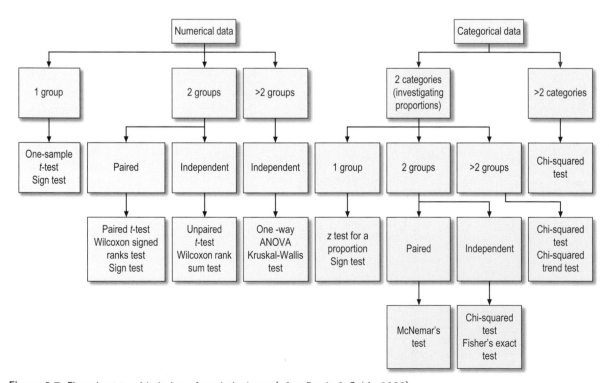

Figure 6.7 Flowchart to aid choice of statistical test (after Petrie & Sabin 2005).

Table 6.7 Goal and data type

Goal	Data type		
	Normal population (parametric) measurement	Non–normal population (non–parametric) rank, score or measurement	Binomial (two possible outcomes)
Describe one group	Mean, standard deviation (SD)	Median, interquartile range	Proportion
Compare one group to a hypothetical value	One-sample t test	–	Chi-square or binomial test
Compare two unpaired groups	Unpaired t test	Wilcoxon two-sample test (Mann–Whitney)	Fisher's test for large samples
Compare two paired groups	Paired t test	Wilcoxon test	McNemar's test
Compare three or more unmatched groups	One-way ANOVA	Kruskal–Wallis test	Chi-square test
Compare three or more matched groups	Repeated – measures ANOVA: • three correlated samples • four correlated samples	Friedman test	Cochrane Q
Quantify association between two variables	Pearson's correlation	Spearman correlation	Contingency coefficients
Predict value from another measured variable	Simple linear regression or non-linear regression	Non-parametric regression	Simple logistic regression
Predict value from several measured or binomial variables	Multiple linear regression or multiple non-linear regression	–	Multiple logistic regression

relationship between ordinal variables, then you should use Spearman's rho. Similarly, if you wanted to look at the relationship of nominal variables, then a chi-square test should be used. It is not the purpose of this book to explore each of the statistical tests in turn: there are numerous texts on the market that provide this information but what is important is that you can identify which tests should be performed so that you can tell when reading a paper whether the correct analysis has been used. A simple flowchart is provided in Figure 6.7, however, just to indicate the broad statistical methods that are available to all.

CONCLUSION

Research design is concerned with the development of a plan for conducting a research study. Many decisions are involved, ranging from definition of the population of interest, the sampling technique, the measurement instrument and the research design to the method of analysis. Errors are possible at each stage, and in reality each study will involve some compromises forced by, for example, time, economic or ethical factors. However, whenever a compromise becomes necessary it is vital to establish exactly why it was necessary and the influence on the data obtained.

KEY CONCEPT

Research in perspective

Every piece of research involves some element(s) of compromise. Whilst the research consumer must identify these and consider their impact on the results obtained, the researcher must identify them at the design stage and ensure that the research design can 'control' for them, i.e. account for them in the results so that their influence does not taint the results.

REFERENCES

Bennett P, Patterson C, Wearing S, Baglioni T 1998 Development and validation of a questionnaire designed to measure foot-health status. J Am Podiatr Med Assoc 88:419–428

Black D 1998 The limitations of evidence. J R Coll Physicians Lond 32:23–26

Bowling A 2004 Measuring disease: a review of disease-specific quality of life measurement scales. Open University Press, London

Bristow I, Dean T 2003 Evidence-based practice – its origins and future in the podiatry profession. Br J Podiatry 6:43–47

Chambers Dictionary 1998 Chambers Harrap, Edinburgh

Chou LH 2006 Reliability and validity of physical examinations. In: Malanga GA, Nadler SF (eds) Musculoskeletal physical examination: an evidence-based approach. Mosby, Philadelphia

Coolican H 2004 Research methods and statistics in psychology, 4th edn. Hodder Arnold, London

Daly L, Bourke G 2000 Interpretation and uses of medical statistics. Blackwell Science, Oxford

de Vet HCW, Terwee CB, Bouter LM 2003 Clinimetrics and psychometrics: two sides of the same coin. J Clin Epidemiol 56:1146–1147

Donaghy M 1999 Reflections on clinical effectiveness in therapy: a practical approach. Br J Ther Rehabil 6:270–274

Farmer R, Miller D, Lawrenson R 1996 Lecture notes on epidemiology and public health medicine. Blackwell Science, Oxford

Feinstein AR 1999 Multi-item 'instruments' vs Virginia Apgar's principles of clinimetrics. Arch Intern Med 159(2):125–128

Giles L 1997 Introduction. In: Giles L, Singer K (eds) Clinical anatomy and management of low back pain, Vol. 1. Butterworth-Heinemann, Oxford

Godlee F 1998 Getting evidence into practice. BMJ 317:50

Gomm R, Needham G, Bullman A 2000 Evaluating research in health and social care. Sage, London

Gordis L 2004 Epidemiology, 3rd edn. WB Saunders, Philadelphia

Greenhalgh T 1996 Is my practice evidence-based? BMJ 313:957–958

Greenhalgh T 2000 How to read a paper: the basics of evidence based medicine, 2nd edn. BMJ Books, London

Greenhalgh T 2006 How to read a paper: the basics of evidence based medicine, 3rd edn. Blackwell Publishing/BMJ Books, Oxford

Hyman GS, Solomon J, Dahm J 2006 Physical examination of the foot and ankle. In: Malanga GA, Nadler SF (eds) Musculoskeletal physical examination: an evidence-based approach. Mosby, Philadelphia

Kilmartin TE, Barrington RL, Wallace WA 1994 A controlled prospective trial of a foot orthosis for juvenile hallux valgus. J Bone Joint Surg-B 76(2):210–214

Kirkwood B, Sterne J 2003 Medical statistics. Blackwell Science, Oxford

Kline P 2000 Handbook of psychological testing. Routledge, London

Kuhn TS 1996 The structure of scientific revolutions, 3rd edn. Chicago University Press, Chicago

Marx RG, Bombardier C, Hogg-Johnson S, Wright JG 1999 Clinimetric and psychometric strategies for development of a health measurement scale. J Clin Epidemiol 52:105–111

Miettinen O 1998 Evidence in medicine: invited commentary. Can Med Assoc J 158:215–221

Morgan DL 1988 Focus groups as qualitative research. Sage, Newbury Park, CA

Murphy K, Davidshoffer C 2005 Psychological testing: principles and application. Pearson Education International, Upper Saddle River, NJ

Petrie A, Sabin C 2005 Medical statistics at a glance. Blackwell Publishing, Oxford

Pickering G 1956 Quote in BMJ:113–116

Pickering G 1956 Cited in Straus S, Richardson WS, Glasziou P, Haynes R 2005 Evidence based medicine: how to practice and teach EBM 3rd edn. Churchill Livingstone, Edinburgh

Polgar S, Thomas S 2000 Introduction to research in the health sciences, 4th edn. Churchill Livingstone, Edinburgh

Rowan K 2001 The development and validation of a multi-dimensions measure of chronic foot pain: the ROwan Foot Pain Assessment Questionnaire (ROFPAQ). Foot Ankle Int 22:795–809

Shapin S 1996 The scientific revolution. University of Chicago Press, Chicago

Streiner DL 2003 Clinimetrics vs. psychometrics: an unnecessary distinction. J Clin Epidemiol 56:1142–1145

Talley N, O'Connor S 1996 Clinical examination. Blackwell Science, Oxford

Upton P, Upton D 2007 The psychometric approach to health-related quality of life measurement: a research users' guide. In: Columbus F (ed) Psychological tests and testing. Nova Science, New York

Vetter NM, Matthews IP 1999 Epidemiology and public health medicine. Churchill Livingstone, Edinburgh

Wald N 1996 The epidemiological approach. In: Souhami R, Moxham J eds Textbook of medicine. Churchill Livingstone, Edinburgh

Wolfs F 2006 Introduction to the scientific method. University of Rochester, NY

Wotruba TR, Wright PL 1975 How to develop a teacher-rating instrument: a research approach. J Higher Educ 46(6):653–663

Chapter 7

Don't lose it, use it!

When the facts change, I change my mind. What do you do?

John Maynard Keynes

LEARNING OUTCOMES

By the end of this chapter you will be able to:

- Discuss the major issues concerning the transfer of research evidence into clinical practice
- Describe the conditions that evidence should satisfy prior to changing practice
- Discuss the methods by which change should be introduced into clinical practice

- Confidently modify your practice in an appropriate way in response to published information.

Case Study

A clinician commonly encounters patients suffering with Achilles tendinopathy. A literature review reveals that numerous conservative and surgical interventions have been described for this common, chronic and debilitating condition, but there is no obviously superior conservative treatment that should dominate initial treatment of this condition. The clinician's attention is drawn to a review article that details, in a very positive light, the results of several articles that investigated the effect of an eccentric calf muscle training regime (Alfredson 2005). This detailed the results of two studies, the first reporting satisfaction in 14 of 15 subjects at 12 weeks (Alfredson et al 1998) and the second reporting success in 90 of 101 tendons.

The clinician is keen to adopt this technique in clinic immediately. Would it be appropriate to do so?

INTRODUCTION

Evidence-based practice is, quite literally, a method of approaching clinical practice where information is sought regarding potential diagnostic tests or treatments to ensure that the best options are selected. The process is, therefore, firmly grounded in *clinical application*, i.e. it exists exclusively to enhance practice. It is vital that we remember this when we approach the literature: if we are unwilling to actually change what we do clinically, or if we do not know how to instigate changes, then there is little value in critically appraising research. When reading published research reports, we are implicitly asking ourselves the question: 'Would it be justified to change our practice based on this research study?' Note that this question need not relate to a treatment – it relates just as well to diagnostic tests. Numerous issues must be considered when contemplating changes in practice and this chapter will consider some of these, including the factors influencing whether a research study should be used to inform clinical practice and the way that changes in practice should be managed. In doing so, this discussion aims to make the implicit question 'Would it be justified to change our practice?' explicit.

Despite the current emphasis on evidence-based practice, it seems that healthcare professionals are slow to change their clinical approach, even in the face of convincing evidence. For example, Greenhalgh (2006) offers various answers to the question: 'Why are health professionals slow to adopt evidence-based practice?', including the perception of individual clinicians regarding the treatment in question, their experience of it and the support it receives. It is clear, therefore, that no discussion of evidence-based practice is complete without considering the factors influencing whether or not a treatment should be adopted in clinic or the manner in which any changes being applied should be instigated and managed. Without confronting these issues, it is unlikely that engaging in the process of EBP will result in a change in practice.

SOURCES OF INFORMATION TO DRIVE CHANGES IN PRACTICE

Whilst we are charged with personally appraising published research to determine whether it is good enough to influence a change in our practice, it is important that we remember to refer to sources of pre-appraised evidence. Pre-appraised evidence refers to existing systematic reviews or summaries of published research that have already been conducted, and it may well be that the condition we are seeking the most effective treatment for may already have been investigated. The Oxford Centre for Evidence-based Medicine recommends using the National Library for Health (NLH) Guidelines and Pathways Database, or York University's Centre for Reviews and Dissemination searchable database, to track down clinical guidelines relating to the particular conditions and treatments in which we are interested. Both sites permit searches of key databases of pre-appraised evidence such as:

- the Cochrane Database of Systematic Reviews
- the Database of Abstracts of Reviews of Effectiveness (DARE)
- the NHS Economic Evaluation Database (NHS EED)
- the Health Technology Assessment database (HTA).

These databases are dominated by information of relevance to medicine, and indeed it can seem that EBP is more applicable and easier to practise in the context of general medical practice where evidence seems prolific. For example, searching for information on 'hypertension' results in 413 hits in DARE and 1056 hits in all between DARE, HTA and NHS EED. Whilst a search for topics of relevance to the practising podiatrist is highly unlikely to yield this number of results, it is nonetheless common to find useful information. For example, DARE contains guidelines concerning the use of physical therapy and low level laser therapy for Achilles tendinopathy, physical interventions for patellofemoral pain syndrome, plantar heel pain, onychomycosis and hallux valgus. Therefore, when faced with new evidence in the form of a research article that we are considering using as a basis for modifying our practice, it is important in the first instance to review existing guidelines. This need not be an onerous task: in exploring the question, 'Can clinicians actually practice EBP?', Straus et al (2005) suggested that if summaries of evidence are prepared and taken to clinic, or when electronic access to pre-appraised data is possible in clinic, they can be accessed in under a minute. Further, and more importantly, it was also found that when junior members of staff – who are more likely to be unsure of what to do – access such information, it changed 25% of their diagnostic and treatment suggestions and added to a further 23% of them. It is not only junior members of staff who should be accessing evidence, however: a recent investigation into the treatment of patellofemoral pain syndrome and Achilles tendinopathy found that the practitioners involved employed an evidence-based approach to practice in only 50% of cases (Murray et al 2005). This suggests that all clinicians should be vigilant in ensuring that their practice techniques are driven by evidence.

However, whilst pre-appraised evidence is ideal for instilling confidence that we are practising according to the best available evidence, the decision on changing practice is more difficult where the 'evidence' is a single research article. This article may be recently published and focus on a test, therapy or condition that is not considered in a pre-appraised review. It may even detail a successful response to a treatment considered by a pre-appraised review to be unsupported. In such situations there is a clear need for guidance to help decide whether it is justified to modify practice. Numerous factors influence the decision to modify our practice and each warrants independent consideration if clinicians are to modify their practice with confidence. These factors include:

- what actually constitutes convincing evidence
- the nature of the condition being treated, including its natural history
- the nature of the intervention
- the consistency of the evidence with existing knowledge
- the patients being treated.

CLINICAL TIP

Implementing the results of our appraisal, step 1

The first step towards incorporating evidence into practice is to have access to good-quality evidence in a clinical setting.

Gathering relevant evidence from, or organizing electronic access to, NLH or the York Centre for Reviews and Dissemination, and making this available in clinic, can provide real-time access to quality information capable of impacting on the care we provide.

WHAT CONSTITUTES CONVINCING EVIDENCE?

Different types or strengths of evidence can be convincing depending on the situation. Single articles are unlikely to provide convincing evidence by

CLINICAL TIP

Implementing the results of our appraisal, step 2

Changes in practice are rarely driven by individual articles. They are driven by a body of evidence that includes multiple different types of study.

If we read about a new technique in one article we must explore it and the underlying rationale further, prior to making a decision regarding whether to incorporate it in clinic.

themselves, and the notion that individual randomized controlled trials (RCTs) will come along that have to be evaluated to make critical decisions regarding clinical treatments undermines the true nature of what we refer to as 'evidence'. Epidemiologists remind us that RCTs and evaluations of treatment have a special place in what is a research *process* (Vetter & Matthews 1999, Gordis 2004). This issue was considered in Chapter 5 which described how single case studies alert us to a particular possibility which is then investigated more formally using designs such as case-control and cohort studies, supported by laboratory research regarding, for example, mechanisms of action. An RCT, therefore, represents the culmination of a programme of research which considers the incidence, prevalence and distribution of a condition, and the factors significantly associated with its onset, which drives the choice of therapy tested by the RCT. As Black (1998) reminds us, evidence is derived from many sources including epidemiological, laboratory and basic science studies, and we are most often convinced by the balance of probabilities than the iron laws of evidence-based practice. This conveys a very important message – if we are considering altering our practice on the basis of a single article, then it is highly probable that we have not sought further evidence so that the article may be considered in the context of the body of evidence that likely exists.

THE NATURE OF THE CONDITION BEING TREATED

An important determinant of the evidence we require before considering changing our practice is the nature of the condition being treated. For example, it is critical that a cardiac surgeon performing coronary bypass surgery, a rheumatologist using biological agents or a psychiatrist treating schizophrenia identifies thoroughly convincing evidence – in the form of a clearly superior technique that is supported by robust statistical data – prior to modifying their practice. This is because the consequences of getting it wrong can be dire, and likely to manifest with substantial morbidity/mortality. Although potentially serious consequences may be associated with modifications to treatment approaches to the diabetic foot or matrix destruction techniques in nail surgery, podiatric pathologies generally carry a lower risk of such consequences. The introduction of new treatments is, therefore, generally associated with fewer risks for many podiatric pathologies. For example, various conservative therapies are recommended for plantar fasciitis, with no clearly superior intervention, and the integration of a new conservative technique that is supported by moderate evidence could be justified. However, this brings us to the next issue that warrants consideration – the intervention being contemplated.

CLINICAL TIP

Make sure you are aware of the potential consequences of any treatment prior to using it. This is not just good practice, it is a legal requirement.

THE NATURE OF THE INTERVENTION

Podiatrists, and a majority of healthcare professionals, are concerned with the treatment of a range of pathologies, and this demands access to a range of interventions. Just as the nature of the condition being treated is important, so too is the nature of the intervention, and for the same reasons: whilst some interventions are highly specialist, others can be safely implemented by patients themselves. For example, it is clearly

CLINICAL TIP

Thinking of incorporating a new technique in your clinical practice? Make sure you understand the exact protocol and are applying the right treatment, to the right patients, with the right presentation of the disorder.

vital that potential modifications to the type of orthoses provided to neuroischaemic diabetic patients be very carefully considered, whilst modifications to a stretching regime require less supporting evidence. This is not to undermine the role of stretching and the potential for consequences should it be performed inappropriately, but it is clearly inappropriate to rank the potential for complications associated with these two interventions as similar. Therefore, when we are considering incorporating a new treatment approach, it is important that we consider the intervention and the potential consequences of its inappropriate use.

Following on from considering the potential consequences associated with a treatment, we must also ensure that we understand and apply the treatment correctly. For example, if a new chemical is being used for matrix destruction, then we must apply it according to the described protocol.

THE CONSISTENCY OF THE EVIDENCE WITH EXISTING KNOWLEDGE

As mentioned, it is highly unlikely that a research paper we read will deal with a totally revolutionary treatment that has not been investigated at all. It is likely that there are reports, discussions, conference proceedings or observational studies related to either the treatment or the causal factor the treatment is attempting to address. It is important that we perform a literature search to uncover this information. If this new and seemingly improved treatment looks considerably worrisome, or is tackling a factor that does not seem to be strongly associated with the disorder being treated, then we should be reluctant to use it. Greenhalgh (2006) provided some useful information with respect to consistency of information, reminding us that all is not always what it seems (Box 7.1), and that asking questions when presented with 'evidence' can be very useful.

Box 7.1 Don't be fooled by misinformation – see through to the vital information!

- Don't listen to a pre-rehearsed sales pitch regarding an intervention.
- Don't fall for the information provided in promotional leaflets/booklets, which are likely to provide unpublished material, misleading graphs (look at the scales) and selective quotations. Ask for results from randomized controlled trials or other useful studies that have been published in peer-reviewed journals.
- Don't be impressed just because a 'celebrity' in your field is using the technique.
- Use the 'STEP' acronym to focus on vital information concerning:
  - **S**afety: What are the indications, contraindications and special precautions?
  - **T**olerability: Do patients comply with this treatment?
  - **E**fficacy: How does the technique/treatment compare with your current choice?
  - **P**rice: How expensive is it, taking into consideration the duration of treatment necessary and the volume of product required for a course of treatment?
- Ensure that claimed benefits (e.g. a longer drug half-life) translate into a clinical benefit. A useful example is in relation to a wound dressing.
- 'New' does not necessarily mean 'better'. Robust evidence is required.

Adapted from *How to get evidence out of a drug rep* (Greenhalgh 2006).

THE PATIENTS BEING TREATED

This issue is undoubtedly already considered by a majority of practitioners and relates to the demands of the individual patients we meet. 'Best' is a relative term when considering treatments and varies considerably from patient to patient. Nail avulsion with phenolization may perhaps be considered the 'best' treatment for nail surgery, but in the high-risk patient the wound resulting from incisional nail surgery is associated with a more rapid healing time and is therefore the 'best' treatment for the high-risk patient. Similarly, a professional footballer whose livelihood depends on activity may also prefer incisional nail surgery as the return to training and competitive play is faster. Patient values and requirements are recognized as essential components of evidence-based practice, and this has two implications:

1. We must ensure that the 'best' treatment is selected with specific reference to the particular patient we are treating.
2. We have a duty to ensure that if there is a new treatment available which is associated with more positive results, we educate ourselves to offer it.

MANAGING CHANGES IN PRACTICE

Conceptually, a desire to practise according to evidence-based principles is an expression of a clinician's desire to do the best they can for their patients. Important lessons about how we should go about adopting a truly evidence-based approach can be learned by considering what the enthusiastic clinician can find themselves doing if not conscientious and discriminating. For example, Greenhalgh (2006) explains how her enthusiasm upon qualification led her to practise by 'press cutting'. This involved amassing useful hints and tips from journal articles which seemed relevant. However, this is a random approach to practice that employs no quality appraisal and is likely to see many ongoing (erratic?) modifications to practice. Similarly, it is tempting to modify our practice based on words of wisdom uttered by distinguished colleagues, although, yet again, there is no quality control involved and practice is not being influenced in a systematic and managed manner. It is clear that changes in practice must be managed in a more rigorous manner, for two reasons: firstly, it is important to ensure that changes in practice take place only when it is appropriate to do so; secondly, we must put in place mechanisms whereby the effectiveness of any changes can be evaluated.

If the effect of a change in practice is to be appreciated, then it is vital that we understand our current effectiveness, otherwise we will have only subjective judgements by which to evaluate practice and such estimates are unlikely to be accurate. It is therefore logical that we must understand our current effectiveness and use this information as a baseline from which to measure the benefit of changes to our practice. The topic of audit is considered in Chapter 8, describing the methodology by which we can establish our baseline performance and, from there, the

CLINICAL TIP

The effect of any modification must be evaluated to determine its benefit. Therefore, understanding our existing effectiveness is vital as it serves as the baseline from which to measure the effect of changes in practice.

effectiveness of any changes to practice. When we are considering changing our practice a specific process should be followed:

1. We should base the decision to change our practice on convincing information – not just from one article.
2. We should audit our existing performance to help us understand where we can improve, and to provide a baseline from which to measure the impact of changes in practice.
3. We should change our practice in a systematic manner – meaning that we do not randomly apply a new treatment to individuals we think are suitable. Rather, we should formulate criteria for the use of a new approach and use the modified treatment whenever indicated by the criteria.
4. We should audit our outcomes so that we know definitively whether the change to our practice resulted in better patient outcomes. This then tells us whether we should adopt the new technique as the standard.

An example drawing all these concepts together concerns the treatment of plantar fasciitis. NeLH Guidelines Finder identifies a treatment algorithm (Thomas et al 2001) for the management of plantar fasciitis which includes the use of stretches for the gastrocnemius and soleus muscles. A literature review identifies a number of articles presenting information supporting this treatment. For example, Riddle et al (2003) conducted a case control study (discussed previously) which identified that subjects with <0° dorsiflexion were 23.3 times more likely to have plantar fasciitis than those with >10°; Kilmartin (1999) found that tension night splints which held the ankle in a dorsiflexed position resulted in cure within 6 months of use in patients with recalcitrant plantar heel pain. In addition, Cheung et al (2006) constructed a model which suggested that with a consistent vertical load applied to the tibia, increasing Achilles tendon load resulted in increasing strain on the plantar fascia, providing a plausible mechanism by which tight posterior muscles may be associated with plantar fascia trauma. All of these studies support the provision of advice on stretches for patients with plantar fasciitis. However, recent studies report on the initial (DiGiovanni et al 2003) and 2-year (DiGiovanni et al 2006) results associated with the addition of tissue-specific plantar fascia stretches to the standard stretching protocol. Results revealed a significantly improved outcome amongst patients who used traditional and plantar fascia stretches, with 'worst pain' and 'first-step pain' both significantly reduced. Should you now provide advice to all patients with plantar fasciitis to include a plantar fascia-specific stretch into their programme? The study focused on subjects with chronic plantar fasciitis, and patients do require some flexibility to be able to self-administer the stretches. However, the stretches are relatively easy to perform, carry limited risk of adverse consequences and seem to be associated with better outcomes. Therefore, after evaluating baseline success with the current regime, using first-step pain and worst pain, it seems reasonable to suggest these stretches to all patients who are physically capable of doing them. Modifying advice for a 3-month period, after which first-step pain and worst pain are evaluated once more, will provide information on the benefits of fully adopting this additional intervention.

CASE STUDY REVISITED

Eccentric training for Achilles tendinopathy

The prospect of a success rate of around 90% in chronic Achilles tendinopathy is enticing. An OVID search reveals that numerous articles have been published concerning eccentric training. This shows that Alfredson's team has been investigating this technique, which comprises painful stretches, since 1998 when a programme involving three sets of 15 heel drops performed daily for 12 weeks resulted in apparent cure in 14 of 15 patients (Alfredson et al 1998). Subsequent larger studies involved the use of the same programme in 78 patients with 101 affected tendons which resulted in 'satisfactory' results in 89% of tendons. These figures relate explicitly to patients with chronic mid-portion Achilles tendinopathy, as application to patients with insertional Achilles tendinopathy, in the same study, resulted in poorer results, with only 32% reporting satisfaction (Fahlstrom et al 2003). Further, comparison of eccentric and concentric programmes suggests the eccentric to be the superior intervention. This information strongly suggests that a 12-week programme of painful eccentric heel drops, comprising three sets of 15 performed twice a day, is the clinical answer to chronic tendinopathy.

However, Sayana and Maffulli (2007) repeated this study in the UK on a sample of 34 sedentary patients and found that after a 12-week training programme 15 (44%) showed no improvement and went on to receive either peritendinous injections or surgery. This information represents something of a quandary for the clinician. What is the truth regarding the effectiveness of eccentric training?

This situation is common: a treatment option appears to be associated with excellent results upon first consideration, before more contentious results are identified and controversy develops. However, using the principles outlined in this chapter can help resolve the dilemma.

Achilles tendinopathy is a common, chronic condition that is difficult to treat. A literature review on the topic reveals that a considerable number of articles have been written on the subject and eccentric heel drops do seem to be a reasonable treatment option. This is because they are associated with a success rate of between 50 and 90%, which, despite the range, offers a fair opportunity of improvement for minimal cost and at minimal inconvenience or pain to the patient. However, drawing the conclusion that 'eccentric heel drops are useful for treating Achilles tendinopathy' is inadequate. There is vital information available in the literature, making the following conclusion more appropriate:

Eccentric heel drops, involving three sets of 15 targeting both the gastrocnemius and soleus muscles, performed twice a day for 12 weeks, with the use of increasing loads as required to ensure that the exercises remain painful throughout the programme, is a potentially useful treatment approach in patients with non-insertional mid-portion tendinopathy. The approach is most likely to be successful in active (versus sedentary) patients.

Therefore, the clinician should confidently use the approach in athletic individuals presenting with mid-portion Achilles tendinopathy, but should take the time to produce patient information leaflets, detailing the specific training programme described in the literature, to improve concordance. The use of the programme in sedentary patients and in those with insertional tendinopathy may be beneficial, but is less likely to be so.

CONCLUSION

It can be very tempting to modify our practice indiscriminately when we learn of a new test or treatment that seems to be associated with good outcomes. However, a reactionary approach which sees many uncontrolled changes to practice sees similar patients treated in different ways and we can be left with a blurred picture of the effectiveness of our interventions. It is vital that when we are considering changes to practice that these are based on robust information, analysis of the condition and the patient being treated, and the intervention being considered. Furthermore, it is crucial that modifications to practice are not applied in a random, reactionary manner where, although trying to do our best for our patients, practice is modified frequently with no ongoing evaluation that allows us to understand the effect of each change.

Chapter 8 will consider audit, a topic concerned with the systematic and objective assessment of performance. Knowledge of audit is invaluable because it shows us how to establish our baseline effectiveness, and helps us to manage changes to practice in a systematic manner and evaluate our subsequent effectiveness.

REFERENCES

Alfredson H 2005 Conservative management of Achilles tendinopathy: new ideas. Foot Ankle Clin 10:321–329

Alfredson H, Pietila T, Jonsson P, Lorentzon R 1998 Heavy load eccentric calf muscle training for the treatment of chronic Achilles tendinosis. Am J Sports Med 26(3):360–366

Black D 1998 The limitations of evidence. J R Coll Physicians Lond 02:20 26

Cheung JT, Zang M, An KN 2006 Effect of Achilles tendon loading on plantar fascia tension in the standing foot. Clin Biomech 21(2):194 203

DiGiovanni B, Nawoczenski D, Lintal M et al 2003 Tissue-specific plantar fascia stretching exercise enhances outcomes in patients with chronic heel pain. J Bone Joint Surg 85A:1270–1277

DiGiovanni B, Nawoczenski D, Malay D et al 2006 Plantar fascia-specific stretching exercise improves outcomes in patients with chronic plantar fasciitis: a prospective clinical trial with two year follow up. J Bone Joint Surg 88A:1775–1781

Fahlstrom M, Jonsson P, Lorentzon R, Alfredson H 2003 Chronic Achilles tendon pain treated with eccentric calf-muscle training. Knee Surg Sports Traumatol Arthrosc 11:327–333

Gordis L 2004 Epidemiology, 3rd edn. WB Saunders, Philadelphia

Greenhalgh T 2006 How to read a paper: the basics of evidence based medicine, 3rd edn. Blackwell Publishing/BMJ Books, Oxford

Kilmartin T 1999 Tension night splints for the treatment of recalcitrant heel pain. Br J Podiatry 2.17–20

Murray IR, Murray SA, MacKenzie K, Coleman S, Cullen M 2005 How evidence based is the management of two common sports injuries in a sports injury clinic? Br J Sports Med 39:912–916

Riddle DL, Pulisic M, Pidcoe P, Johnson RE 2003 Risk factors for plantar fasciitis: a matched case-control study. J Bone Joint Surg 85A:872–877

Sayana M, Maffulli N 2007 Eccentric calf muscle training in non-athletic patients with Achilles tendinopathy. J Sci Med Sport 10(1):52–58

Straus S, Richardson WS, Glasziou P, Haynes R 2005 Evidence-based medicine: how to practice and teach EBM 3rd Ed. Churchill Livingstone, Edinburgh

Thomas JL, Christenson JC, Kravitz SR et al 2001 Clinical practice guideline: the diagnosis and treatment of heel pain. J Foot Ankle Surg 40(5):329–340

Vetter NM, Matthews IP 1999 Epidemiology and public health medicine. Churchill Livingstone, Edinburgh

Chapter 8

What difference does it make?

What you do speaks so loud that I cannot hear what you are saying.
Ralph Waldo Emerson

LEARNING OUTCOMES

By the end of this chapter you will be able to:
- Define audit and highlight its importance in everyday clinical practice
- Discuss the difference between research and audit
- Discuss the links between research and audit
- Explore the elements of the audit cycle
- Be aware of the process necessary to complete an audit.

INTRODUCTION

CLINICAL TIP

Everyone should be involved in clinical audit – it is part of the clinical governance framework.

CLINICAL TIP

Everyone in your practice may be involved in audit: don't forget the support and administrative staff!

Up to this point the chapters have focused on the early steps of the research process: the specification of your research question, the literature search to refine your question and the methods used in addressing your question. However, is this where the process stops? Of course not: the aim of any applied health research is to improve the care for the patient or client by improving diagnosis, intervention or service delivery. However, how do we know if the changes we have instigated on the basis of our critical appraisal of the literature have been of any value? How do we know whether the changes we have made have been successful and achieved what we want? In short, have we made a positive difference to the experience of the patient?

The process of audit is designed to help us determine just how effective our current practice, or any change in practice, is, and is something that all healthcare professionals should be familiar with and engaged in.

In this chapter we will explore the issue of audit – asking, and answering, several key questions: What is audit? How does it relate to, and differ from, research? What are the processes involved in research and audit? How should podiatrists undertake audit? Should the two processes be considered separately or do we need to integrate them? Are there skills relating to research that we can use in audit and vice-versa?

Case Study

The NHS service at the local Michael Flatley Foot Clinic has decided to audit the interactions between podiatrists and their older adult clients. The Flatley Clinic is an NHS-run clinic that accepts routine referrals from a variety of sources: each podiatrist has a heavy clinical workload. In addition, the Clinic has a large intake of podiatry students on placement. This being the case, there are a relatively high number of recent graduates working at the Clinic. However, these recruits tend not to stay too long and often move on to jobs outside of the inner-city environment in which the Clinic is based. The Flatley Clinic is well known in the local area and has close links with the nearby university. It has a specialism in the older adult and these form the majority of their cases.

The clinical staff considered there to be a few problems with communication and it was decided that an audit in this area should take place. They considered a clinical audit of patient communication to be important because both government and local managers have emphasized the importance of 'patient satisfaction' as a quality indicator. Furthermore, patient satisfaction correlates with satisfaction in other aspects of contact – in particular, adherence to treatment.

The Flatley Clinic podiatrists selected this topic for audit for three clear reasons:

- Podiatrists early in their career and those on placement can be somewhat anxious about seeing patients for the first time and they wanted some feedback on how the patients saw them.

- Nobody at the Clinic had reviewed the views of patients previously.
- Research has indicated that the quality of the initial patient contact can influence adherence to treatment.

The aim of the staff when completing this audit was to establish *standards* of the first contact of the podiatrist with the older adult and how well these standards were being met. The standards define the aspect of care to be measured, and should always be based on the best available evidence. A standard is the threshold of the expected compliance for each criterion (these are usually expressed as a percentage). A criterion is a measurable outcome of care, aspect of practice or capacity.

WHY AUDIT?

During the preceding 20 years or so the framework of podiatric care (and health in general) has changed greatly, with considerable emphasis now being centred on (as we have previously stressed) evidence-based practice and clinical effectiveness. This has led to considerable changes in the organization and delivery of the health service and the culture in which podiatrists operate (Trinder & Reynolds 2000). One such change has been the introduction of clinical audit which involves using techniques and standards to improve service to patients.

Crombie et al (1993) suggest that the need for clinical audit may occur because of some of the following explanations.

- *The differences in the care provided*: There may be quite significant differences in the delivery of care from institution to institution or from country to country. At the outset, it may be impossible to determine what form of provision is best but the audit may help to determine this – or at least if one method or process is better than another.
- *Limitation of resources*: In these days of finite resources it is essential that those available are used to their best effect. Obviously, an audit may help guide the use of resources.
- *Evident deficiencies in the care delivered*: Audit can demonstrate if there are any deficiencies in the delivery of care.

CLINICAL TIP

Conducting an audit can provide your manager with the evidence required to facilitate change. This may include securing further funds, more staff and other resources.

- *Organizational need for audit*: The quality of work can be monitored within an organization through audit.
- *Technological advances and professional education*: New technology or professional education can be used to help remedy any deficits in the care provided.
- *Political power of audit*: If any weaknesses are identified then this evidence can be used to monitor and change behaviours/processes.

Clinical audit has as its goal the improvement of clinical activity: it compares actual practice to a standard of practice and any deficiencies in actual practice can thus be identified and rectified. In this way there should be improved outcomes for patients. There are a number of benefits of a good, reliable audit which include:

- substantial improvements in the quality of service to patients
- improved communication between disciplines, professions and at the primary/secondary care interface
- being a valuable educational tool
- helping to highlight and prioritize key issues and problems
- preventing problems recurring
- better overall utilization of resources
- improving morale.

The process of clinical audit has been strongly promoted within the NHS, and although many surveys have demonstrated that the majority of clinicians have attempted clinical audit, many audits are not completed (Shakib & Phillips 2003), the common barriers being lack of support and supervision, difficulties with data collection and a perceived lack of time. Thus, at the outset, the following should be emphasized: audit is important for patient care, but there are obstacles and barriers that you will face; be prepared, and prepare yourself by gaining support for your audit. This may be in the form of a time allowance, or administrative or technical help with gathering and processing data.

KEY CONCEPT

Clinical audit has as its aim the improvement of patient care.

WHAT IS AUDIT?

An accepted definition of clinical audit is 'a quality improvement process that seeks to improve patient care and outcomes through systematic review of care against explicit criteria and the implementation of change' (NICE 2002). Although there are many definitions of audit, several have the following characteristics for the podiatrist:

- The patient is the major focus of the audit and should benefit from it.
- It is systematic based on measurable standards.

- There are clearly identifiable professionals or groups of professionals that take responsibility for the audit.
- The audit relates to the podiatrist's own patients.
- The results, where indicated, lead to positive change in the care of patients.

There are a number of types of audit: peer review, adverse occurrence screening, patient satisfaction survey, critical incident monitoring and criterion-based audit. The methods involved in these types of audit obviously differ but what is common is that they all involve the collection of some form of data – whether this is through a survey or collation of routinely collected clinical data.

KEY CONCEPT

All audits involve some form of data collection.

SIMILARITIES BETWEEN AUDIT AND RESEARCH

From the description provided so far, surely there is overlap between audit and research? Aren't we simply describing the same process, but using a different term? Indeed, there are some clear similarities between audit and research:

- Audit and research involve answering specific questions relating to quality of care.
- Audit and research can be carried out either prospectively or retrospectively.
- Both involve careful sampling, design and analysis.
- Both have to be professional in terms of leadership and conduct.

CLINICAL TIP

Do not treat research as audit, or audit as research.

CLINICAL TIP

Audit is not just a backdoor approach to research. Take the time to understand the characteristics of each.

Although many may argue that there is no difference between audit and research and the differences that do exist are minor and of minimal relevance, this is not the case. The distinction between the two is important – especially given the ubiquitous Research Governance Framework (DH 2001) which we will explore in more detail in Chapter 9. Healthcare professionals, however, may treat the two as synonymous for these reasons, along with something more pragmatic: because of the introduction of research governance it is now much more difficult, time-consuming and frustrating to get approval for any research. Consequently, there is an attraction to try to get projects classified as 'audit topics' rather than 'research' in order to bypass the processes (Jones & Bamford 2004, Smith 2000, Watson & Manthorpe 2002).

Many clinicians faced with the research governance processes and the requirements to go through scientific scrutiny committees and ethics committees have asked themselves or their colleagues: 'Can we call this audit and avoid the hassle of these forms and committees?' Kneafsey and

Task

Consider a clinical audit activity related to your practice – what research skills and activities will be required in order to undertake it?

Howarth (2004) argue that there will be an increase in so-called 'audit activity' in the current atmosphere of the research governance framework. This can be problematic, of course, since it means that some current audits and some audit proposals will not get reviewed through the research governance processes even though they would benefit from so doing. Many researchers see the research governance process as an impediment to research, but it should not be seen in this way. It should be seen as a positive, two-way process that can benefit your research, your practice and the service delivery (more information on research governance is provided in Chapter 9).

DIFFERENCES BETWEEN AUDIT AND RESEARCH

Task

Consider the case study presented earlier. Using the definitions in Table 8.1, demonstrate how it can be described as an audit rather than research. Complete an extra column highlighting how this can be the case. Where are there points of debate?

There are clear differences between audit and research (www.ubht. nhs.uk, 2006) (Box 8.1). *Research* is about creating new knowledge; knowledge about whether new treatments work and whether certain treatments work better than others. In essence we can consider that research forms the basis of our nationally agreed clinical guidelines and standards – it determines what best practice is. *Clinical audit*, on the other hand, is a way of finding out whether we are doing what we should be doing. As Smith (1992) points out: 'Research is concerned with discovering the right thing to do; audit with ensuring that it is done right' (and, of course, clinical effectiveness is about the dissemination of 'the right thing to do' and getting it into practice). Although audit and non-experimental research may have common characteristics, Cooper and Benjamin (2004) highlight the difference clearly: 'The distinction is in their intention [...] As a general rule, clinical audit ensures we achieve the outcomes that have been agreed in set standards; research provides new knowledge and the evidence on which to base such standards.'

The differences, more specifically, are presented in Table 8.1.

Box 8.1 Definitions – audit and research

- *Audit:* The systematic critical analysis of the quality of medical care, including the procedures used for diagnosis and treatment, the use of resources and the resulting outcome and quality of life for the patient (DH 1989).

- *Research:* Rigorous and systematic enquiry conducted on a scale and using methods commensurate with the issues investigated and designed to lead to generalizable contributions to knowledge (DH 1993).

A SIMPLE TEST TO TELL THE DIFFERENCE

There are three simple questions that you could use to determine whether you are conducting audit or research, and if you can follow Figure 8.1 through, then you should be able to find out whether you are doing (or planning) an audit.

Table 8.1 The differences between research and audit

Research	Audit
Creates new knowledge about what works and what doesn't	Answers the question, 'Are we following best practice?'
Is based on hypothesis	Measures against standards
Is usually carried out on a large scale over a prolonged period	Is usually carried out on a relatively small population over a short time span
May involve patients receiving a completely new treatment	Never involves a completely new treatment
May involve experiments on patients	Never involves anything being done to patients beyond their normal clinical management. (Although patient surveys could be construed as 'doing something to patients', it is important that these are designed to be minimally intrusive.)
May involve patients being allocated to different treatment groups	Never involves allocation of patients to different treatment groups
Is based on a scientifically valid sample size (although this may not apply to pilot studies)	Depending on circumstances, may be pragmatically based on a sample size which is acceptable to senior clinicians
Extensive statistical analysis of data is routine	Some statistical analysis may be useful. (Simple descriptive statistics (e.g. mean, median and mode) may be a routine part of audit; more complex analysis (inferential statistics) is not always necessary.)
Results are generalizable and hence publishable	Results are only relevant within local setting (although audit process may be of interest to wider audience and hence audits are also published)
Responsibility to act on findings is unclear	Responsibility to act on findings rests with clinical directorate(s)
Findings influence the activities of clinical practice as a whole	Findings influence activities of local clinicians and teams
Always requires ethics approval	Does not require ethics approval. (Although patient surveys could be considered as part of a research process, it is important that surveys are designed and conducted in such a manner as to cause minimal disruption to patients. Obviously it is worth checking whether your survey requires ethical consideration and approval.)

Source: Clinical Audit Central Office (2000).

THE LINK BETWEEN AUDIT AND RESEARCH

From the discussion presented so far it is apparent that there is a link between research and audit and this is recognized in government publications. The National Health Service's Clinical Effectiveness Initiative draws a clear link between clinical audit and research (see Table 8.1). We need research in order to determine what clinically effective practice is; conversely, we need audit to be able to determine whether this research is actually being practised. More specifically,

- Clinical audit should be legitimately perceived as the final stage of a good clinical research programme.
- On the other hand, research can be seen as the first step in the clinical audit process.

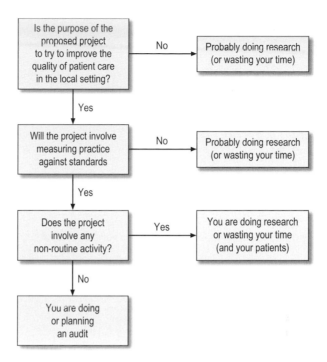

Figure 8.1 Flowchart differentiating between audit and research.

- Research studies are able to help identify areas for audit.
- Audit can highlight deficiencies and where good research evidence is required.
- The audit process can help the promotion of evidence-based practice.

So, for example, research might ask: 'What is the most effective way of treating plantar fasciitis?' and audit would then ask: 'How are we treating plantar fasciitis and how does this compare with accepted best practice?'

Research in this case would involve assessing the outcomes associated with plantar fasciitis and in this way discover the best treatment. Audit, on the other hand, would assess the process (Are we using the outcomes of our research appropriately?) but may also review the outcomes: in this case to review the success of a treatment that we know works, rather than to find out whether it works or how it works (a subtle but important difference). Hence, podiatric research is such that we have clear guidelines for the treatment of certain conditions where we know that these work. In contrast, we have other conditions where we do not know what the most effective treatment is (e.g. plantar fasciitis) and hence cannot monitor, strictly, successful treatment outcomes.

THE AUDIT PROCESS

Typically the audit process is portrayed as a cycle that includes the identification of a problem, the remedy for the problem and the assessment of whether the problem has, indeed, been remedied. As can be seen from

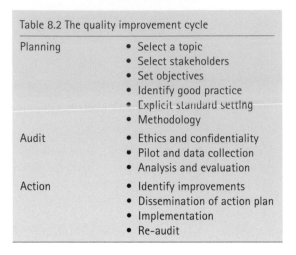

Table 8.2 The quality improvement cycle

Planning	• Select a topic
	• Select stakeholders
	• Set objectives
	• Identify good practice
	• Explicit standard setting
	• Methodology
Audit	• Ethics and confidentiality
	• Pilot and data collection
	• Analysis and evaluation
Action	• Identify improvements
	• Dissemination of action plan
	• Implementation
	• Re-audit

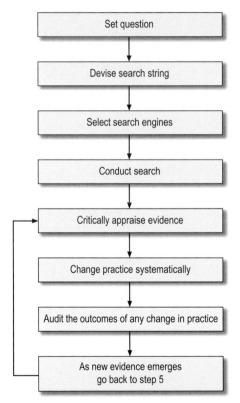

Figure 8.2 Integrating audit into the process of evidence-based practice.

Figure 8.1 and Table 8.2, there are a number of stages and each of these will now be discussed in turn.

However, we can also see how we can integrate audit into evidence-based practice (Fig. 8.2).

We have to remember that if you identify a better way of doing something, instigate a systematic change. Randomly applying evidence blurs

CLINICAL TIP

An audit may require additional resources, including support time and the provision of materials.

its effectiveness. Adopting a change in practice for a trial period (e.g. 3 months) will allow its effect to be audited and compared with the outcomes in the previous 3-month period. It will then be possible to determine whether the 'best evidence' has, in fact, turned out to be 'best' for your patients. This also allows you to justify continuing with the change.

IDENTIFICATION OF THE TOPIC

The first stage in the audit cycle is the identification of the topic to be reviewed. This is best achieved by discussing the issue(s) with colleagues as it is always important to ensure that there is consensus within the service. However, just discussing the issue with colleagues, whilst important, is not sufficient. There must be a clear rationale for this choice and perhaps the following points will help guide the discussion (NICE 2002):

- *Topic of high cost, volume or risk to staff*: It is obvious that the more relevant a topic is for audit the more important it would be to complete.
- *Evidence of serious quality problem*: If there is some indication as to an issue that requires attention in your clinical practice then this should be explored.
- *Is good evidence available to inform standards?*: Since an audit compares against standards then there is a requirement for some standards to be available!
- *Is the problem amenable to change?* An audit always has as its aim the changing and improvement of practice. If the problem is not changeable then there is little purpose in attempting to change it.
- *Is the topic a national policy initiative?*: If an issue has become of national importance then it is more likely to be a relevant and key issue that would be supported by appropriate services.
- *Is the topic a priority for the organization?*: Again, if the topic is relevant and important to the organization then it will be a priority and support will be available.
- *Is the topic a national audit project?*: Some projects will be part of a national project that will be encouraged at a local level.

From this description we can see that there is some overlap with the skills required in researching a particular topic – we have to select carefully, have some good background evidence and clearly articulate the question (see Chapter 3). Answers to the questions will reveal a number of potential audit topics and, of course, there is then a need to rank the topics in terms of a range of factors.

A checklist for making a decision about the topic for an audit should include the following:

- Is it of clinical concern?
- Does it concern service users?
- Is it something of high risk?
- Is it something that happens frequently?
- Does it interest you and your colleagues?
- Does it involve something that is complex or difficult?
- Is it of high cost?
- Are national or professional standards available?

CLINICAL TIP

Before you finalize your decision, ask yourself some common-sense questions:

- Is It Important?
- Is it do-able?
- Is everyone who should be involved, involved?
- Is it ethically sound?

CLINICAL TIP

Do not overstretch yourself. If you are experienced at audit, all well and good. If not, then start small and move onwards and upwards as your experience grows.

There are a number of ways of prioritizing the choice of topic and, of course, it may be derived on the basis of clinician choice (i.e. something that concerns you most) or something that is of high risk (i.e. causing you or your patient potential danger), or it may be a choice based on the frequency of the event. Alternatively, you could decide that the choice be based on the concern of the patient, the evidence available and the cost to the patient. Whatever ranking system you use, however, you should ensure that it is fully agreed by the team before commencing.

An important part of selecting an audit topic is agreement by the team as to the level of evidence that will be required to justify any proposed improvement or change to practice as a result of the study. The Oxford Centre for Evidence-Based Medicine (www.cebm.net) provides details of each level of Sackett's approach, whilst the SIGN guidelines are available at the web address provided in Appendix 1. The concept of changing practice, and the evidence required to convince us that it is appropriate, are considered in Chapter 7.

If we return to our original case study at the Flatley Clinic then we note that the selection of topic was driven by the clinical team in response to a range of pertinent factors: the emphasis on patient satisfaction as an outcome measure, the importance of communication in improving adherence to treatment, the current make-up of the clinic staff and the need to provide an adaptable and quality service to its particular client group. Looking at the checklist we presented earlier:

- *Clinical concern*: Yes, the communication between patients and clinicians was of concern to the service.
- *Concern of service users*: Probably, although this was to be determined by the audit.
- *High risk*: Potential poor adherence to treatment and serious consequences.
- *High volume*: Yes, communication with the patients that formed the majority of the workload was being audited.
- *Clinician interest*: Yes, it was a decision taken by the whole clinical team.
- *Complex or difficult management*: Not really, but did have considerable implications.
- *High cost*: Not really of high cost, but potentially in terms of non-adherence to treatment and continuance of treatment.
- *Availability of national or professional standards*: Very few were in existence.

SELECT STAKEHOLDERS

As highlighted at the outset, the choice of topic should be guided by discussions with colleagues – people need to be on board in order for the audit to be a success. Audit rarely succeeds when performed in isolation and derives positive outcomes from being developed and undertaken by all members of the team, whether from the same professional team or from the multi-disciplinary team. It is important that when designing the audit to link into and work with the existing forums within your organization – these vary from organization to organization but there is usually some form of support for clinical audit. This may not be the case for those in private practice or those working alone: so should they be involved in audit? Well yes, and the special considerations for those working alone are presented in Box 8.2.

Box 8.2 Doing audit when working individually

- Audit your work regularly.
- Remember you may be the only podiatrist but you may not be the only professional working in that service.
- Link with professional colleagues in the locality.
- Select topics that make sense to you, your practice and are manageable.
- Seek support.

The clinical staff involved in delivering care in the organization and related services should be involved as should – of course – people who receive the care or use the service. Ultimately, your practice may be changed (this is the aim of your audit after all) and so you should consider who may be involved in changing practice and who are the key people to influence any changes identified as a result of the audit. These are key stakeholders who should be involved in the audit.

It is also important to note that different people will need to be included at differing stages of the audit cycle. Consequently you have to consider who needs to be informed that the audit is being completed, who should provide the necessary information for the audit, who needs to receive feedback from the audit, and who needs to be included in the planning and carrying out the actions identified by the audit.

Returning to the Flatley Clinic case study, we can see that there are a number of individuals and professions involved – from the podiatrist to the receptionist. All should be involved in the audit as outlined.

EXERCISE

Look at the Flatley Clinic case study – who are the stakeholders and how are they involved at each stage of the audit?

SET CLEAR OBJECTIVES

After selecting a topic it is important for the practitioner or clinical team to agree exactly what is trying to be achieved or established. The audit should concentrate on collecting specific data, using the simplest method in the shortest possible time. You should use the aim as the broad statement of intent, and then break down the audit into components that are measurable and time limited (they should be SMART – see Box 8.3).

Box 8.3 SMART principles

S is for Specific

M is for Measurable

A is for Achievable

R is for Realistic

T is for Timescale

Table 8.3 provides an example of broad questions that have been reduced to specific audit aims.

Table 8.3 Broad questions that have been reduced to specific audit aims

Question	Audit aim
Are we managing elderly people who fall based on best practice standards?	Improve the management of elderly patients who fall
Are we using best practice standards to assess patients with leg ulcers?	Improve the assessment of ambulatory patients with leg ulcers
Are we communicating well with our patients?	Assess the satisfaction of elderly patients when communicating with clinic podiatrists

IDENTIFYING GOOD PRACTICE

Once the subject has been decided, it is key that appropriate standards or criteria against which current practice can be assessed are identified. An essential component of the audit process is the identification of these standards. The standards that are developed should be derived from guidelines (e.g. those produced by NICE) and these standards should (wherever possible) be evidence based. Obviously, the guidelines that you produce should be suited to both your organizational environment and the population under discussion. It is no good applying guidelines derived from a population in a comfortable rural environment to those in a deprived inner-city environment.

Obviously there can be some problems if there are no published standards. If this is the case then they will need to be formulated according to good-quality evidence. There are good sources of literature that can be reviewed in order to derive these guidelines. For example, you may want to consult:

- the evidence-based literature present in journals
- organizational guidelines (e.g. NICE, a podiatry organization or the Health Professions Council)
- expert opinion
- local consensus.

However, with the latter two it should be noted that the same rules apply as when searching the literature: a hierarchy of evidence exists and this should be taken into account when considering the derivation of guidelines (see Chapter 9).

The staff at the Flatley Clinic conducted a literature search using Medline, CINAHL and PsychInfo without much success. A manual search was then undertaken using the *British Journal of Podiatry, The Foot* and the *Journal of the American Podiatric Medical Association*. Very few relevant articles were located and those that were included those by DiMatteo (2004a,b) and Stevenson et al (2004).

EXPLICIT STANDARDS SETTING

The setting of standards is fundamental to the audit process since these explicit standards provide the framework against which practice can be improved. The standards need to be based on SMART guidelines and current research evidence or, if necessary, professional recommendations.

DEVELOPMENT OF METHODOLOGY

At this stage, an appropriate audit methodology must be developed and can include, as we have seen, methods akin to those involved in the research process. At the outset, if we are assessing practice, then the target population along with sample size has to be selected. In Chapter 6 we identified how the sample can be selected if there are a large number of potentially suitable individuals and the audit team must decide on the process of selecting this sample. Obviously we have to ensure that our sample is unbiased (as in research) and is representative of the initial population. Research involves a rigorous sampling strategy, whereas an audit may be based on more practical factors (Clinical Central Audit Office 2000).

Selecting cases

Before you select your audit sample you need to identify the population as clearly as possible since the results you obtain will be applicable only to the population you choose.

The examples provided in Table 8.4 demonstrate how clearly the population has to be defined. For the first example there would be no point in simply saying that the population was 'older people' or for the second 'those with a leg ulcer': this is not clearly defined and the results would not be applicable to these populations.

It may be the case that there is a need to select a sample because the population is large and hence it is impractical to review every patient record or that the timescale is too short; remember, however, that too small a sample may result.

In determining the sample size the requirements of research need not be met. When completing research the sample size should be sufficient for statistical significance (when undertaking quantitative analysis) and credibility since ultimately it must be applicable to a wider population.

Table 8.4 Defining a study population

Example	Study population
To improve the management of elderly people who fall	People of 65 years or over who have fallen and subsequently received inpatient podiatric care and for whom the fall is the key reason for therapy intervention
To improve the management of ambulatory patients with leg ulcers	Patients receiving ambulatory care whose leg ulcers show no improvement for a period of 6 weeks or more
To improve the communication with older people attending the clinic	Patients aged over 60 who are attending the clinic for the first time

There are a range of statistical methods for determining sample size (see Chapter 6) which relate to the 'power' of the analysis. In contrast, when determining the sample size for audit, the sample should be sufficient for gaining commitment to act (i.e. descriptive statistics) and the results need not be generalizable to the population as a whole. However, this does not mean that when completing an audit the sampling technique can be laissez-faire and less robust than when completing a research study. For example, inclusions must be representative of the population from whom they were drawn and the sample selection criteria have to be reviewed and, ultimately, agreed by the complete audit team. Methods for sampling may include the following:

- *Systematic sampling*: Selecting every 5th, 10th, 50th or 100th case, for example, and choosing to start at a random point and then reviewing only those cases that are identified in the sampling.
- *Simple random sampling*: Each person in the population has an equal chance of being drawn. A random number generator is then used to select the sample.
- *Stratified random sampling*: In this case, you may specify the characteristics you wish your sample to have based on the population under discussion. For example, if your population has a 40% ethnic minority proportion, you would select your sample on the basis of having a 40% ethnic sample proportion.

At the Flatley Clinic the sample comprised all new cases attending their first appointment over a 6-month period. Those attending had to be over the age of 60 years and have the necessary reading skills to complete the questionnaire. This was a discrete, and simply described, sample and one that could be easily recruited.

But how can the data be gathered? The team has to decide on the approach to the data collection and these methods can, of course, be akin to those involved in research and is not simply checking case notes (which is the stereotypical view of audit). This array of approaches can include asking questions (using, for example, either a questionnaire or an interview), undertaking an observation study (of typical practice for example) or collecting laboratory samples. Obviously, research investigators use these forms of methods as well as audit. You should ask yourself a series of questions at this stage which are similar to those previously described for research (Box 8.4).

Box 8.4 Questions to ask yourself

- How will I collect the data?
- What level of support will I be offered to collect the data?
- What quantity of data is likely to be generated?
- Can I handle these data?
- Will I need access to spreadsheets, databases or statistical packages?
- Do I have access to this software and can I use it?
- How do I want to present my data?

CLINICAL TIP

Remember not to bias your sample.

Developing an audit tool

There are two fundamental issues that should be addressed at this stage: the selection of cases for audit and the development/selection of the audit instrument.

The audit tool is the basic device for collecting the data and this can be through a number of methods: data capture sheet, questionnaire, interviews and the like. Obviously there are a number of basic questions that need to be asked in order to derive the data collection tool (Box 8.5).

Box 8.5 Basic questions to derive the data collection tool

- What data do you need to collect?
- When will the data be collected – retrospectively or prospectively?
- Who will collect the data?
- Will data collection be manual or electronic?
- What is an appropriate design?
- How will the data collection forms be collated?

You should also consider the following key criteria when developing any data collection form:

- *Validity*: Does your tool accurately measure what you are trying to measure? (See Chapter 6.)
- *Reliability* (see Chapter 6 for further discussion of this concept): Does your tool consistently measure the variables of interest? Would you get the same results if you used the same tool on the same patient, in the same state at different times? (If different people are collecting the same data, then they should have the same results.)
- *Generalizability*: Is the tool you have devised equally applicable to everyone in the designated group?
- *Appropriateness*: Is it appropriate for the purpose you are designing it for?

When you have designed the data collection tool you should check that it does what you hope it does before you start (so you don't waste your, your colleagues' or your patients' time). As a first task you should ask for feedback from colleagues who have not been involved in the process of development: they can check the interpretation of the wording and give feedback on the validity of the tool by questioning the rationale for including or excluding certain items. Furthermore, distributing to colleagues may also publicize your audit.

Once colleagues have commented on the pilot tool it should be piloted on perhaps 10% of the sample (although this is merely a rule of thumb). The results of this pilot study will indicate whether the tool is suitable for meeting the goals of the audit or whether modifications are required.

When undertaking the audit the Flatley Clinic reviewed the literature and concluded that the current questionnaires for gathering patient

Figure 8.3 The Flatley Clinic communication questionnaire.

THE FLATLEY CLINIC COMMUNICATION QUESTIONNAIRE

Instructions to podiatrists/reception staff

Please give every patient aged over 65 years a questionnaire and envelope at the end of your first session. Please explain:

- We are asking people who come to the Flatley Clinic to help us understand what it is like to come here for the first time by filling out this questionnaire.
- We do not need to know anyone's name and all information will be anonymous.
- Please could they fill in the questionnaire in the waiting room, put the sheet in the envelope and post it in the postbox in the waiting room as they leave.
- If anyone would like any help filling the sheet in, please tell the reception staff and they will find someone to help.

Instructions for patients

All those patients who come to the Flatley Podiatric Clinic are being asked to complete a simple questionnaire in order to help us understand more about what it is like to come here for the first time. If you could please answer the following questions that would be extremely useful, and if you could try and answer all the questions. Please be as honest as you can – your name will be included with the questionnaire and the results will be totally confidential.

Please circle word/phrase which best describes the way you feel.

1. How relaxed did you feel during the session you have just had?

Very relaxed	Quite relaxed	Not Sure	Tense	Very Tense

2. Did the podiatrist make it easier or more difficult for you to say what you wanted to say today?

Much easier	Easier	Not sure	More difficult	Very difficult

3. How well do you think your point of view was understood today?

Very well	Quite well	Not sure	Poorly	Very badly

4. Do you think the Flatley Clinic has something to offer you?

Yes, definitely	Probably	Not sure	Probably not	Definitely not

5. How well did you think the podiatrist explained your treatment?

Very well	Quite well	Not sure	Poorly	Very badly

Thank you very much for your help

Please put the sheet in the envelope and post it in the letter box on your way out.

CLINICAL TIP

Although collecting data through self-report is relatively easy, it still requires planning and development.

satisfaction were not suited for this project since they seemed to concentrate on the medical arena rather than the podiatric one. As a result, the audit team of the Flatley Clinic concluded that they should design a self-report questionnaire for the older adult sample. This questionnaire would assess communication satisfaction following the first session.

The questionnaire (Fig. 8.3) consisted of five statements devised using a Likert framework and each of these statements tapped into the standards set, with each statement being followed by five possible responses.

In order to make a sensible comparison the same questionnaire was used by the clinicians. In an attempt to reduce any potential bias in this study (e.g. in terms of the patients wanting to 'look good' or 'give positive feedback'), each of the questionnaires was completed anonymously and patients were requested to fill in the questionnaires following their departure from the clinic, returning them to secretarial or reception staff in envelopes left in the department.

EXERCISE

What do you think of the questionnaire? Evaluate it from an audit and a research perspective.

ETHICS AND CONFIDENTIALITY

Audit is considered a routine part of clinical governance and can be conducted without informed consent and does not usually require ethical approval. However, before assuming you don't require ethical approval, consider (UBHT 2007):

- Is your project really audit?
- Does your project include a patient survey? If so,
  - Are the questions worth asking?
  - Is the choice of a survey appropriate?
  - If contact is to be made with patients away from the clinic, have you taken reasonable steps to ensure that patients are alive?
  - Are the numbers involved sufficient to answer the question?
  - Have the same patients already been targeted for other surveys/research?
  - How will you ensure that patients freely consent to taking part?
  - What written information will be given to patients to explain what the survey is about?
  - How will you ensure patient confidentiality and how will you communicate this to the patients?
  - Will the survey cause minimal disturbance?
  - Will the survey in any way interfere with the treatment of patients?
- Are you planning to publish?

Just because audit does not have to go through an ethics committee does not mean ethical principles can be ignored. Clinical audit must always be conducted within an ethical framework (e.g. doing good and no harm, ensuring confidentiality). In terms of clinical audit you should be aware of the Caldicott principles (DH 2005) and should consider the extent to which patient information needs to be used, the storage of information during the course of the audit and how to ensure that non-identifiable information is used in reports.

PILOT

A pilot study should always be undertaken to ensure that the instrument developed is adequate for the purpose for which it is developed and that the method developed for undertaking the audit actually works. Hence, when the staff at the Flatley Clinic were devising their study, they first completed a pilot study on the questionnaire developed and then tested out the whole process. This was important since it involved the reception staff collecting the questionnaires. At the pilot stage it was realized that the reception staff were becoming overburdened with collecting these when the clinic was busy (and it was causing delays). Consequently, the audit was changed and a 'postbox' was set up so that responders could simply post their completed questionnaires through the letter box and these were collated at the end of the day. This was less of a burden on the reception staff.

ANALYSIS AND EVALUATION

Once the data have been obtained, they must be analysed. This may involve analytical research techniques similar to those discussed previously (see Chapter 6). You must decide how to complete the analysis (by hand or computer). It might be daunting to do it by hand but audit does not require any complicated statistical analyses: no two-way ANOVAs are required! You may also need to call on some form of support and organize this if necessary.

At this stage the differences between audit and research become clearer. Descriptive statistics will usually have to be presented in order to demonstrate the extent to which the standard has, or has not, been met. Data analysis could be calculated, as a rule, by computing compliance rates for each standard: for example, 66% of patients with X have been treated with Y. It is important to analyse your audit data so that an unambiguous, complete, accurate and unbiased view of real-life practice can be provided and that this relates directly to the audit objectives. It is then crucial that results are discussed with colleagues to identify areas that need to be changed.

> **CLINICAL TIP**
>
> Remember to disseminate your results as widely as possible – there may be colleagues elsewhere that would welcome your results.

The data can be presented so that everyone can see the degree to which actual practice is consistent with good practice (i.e. the standards) and, conversely, any shortcomings in practice that may be apparent. Furthermore, a peer review of cases that do not meet the standard will be necessary in order to determine clinically acceptable and unacceptable cases; if there are any unacceptable cases, then the causes of these should be determined.

> **CLINICAL TIP**
>
> Auditing such a topic requires sensitivity – some practitioners may find it threatening.

At the Flatley Clinic, simple bar charts, with percentages of the proportion of patients who responded in each category to the statements, were presented. The results of the investigation are shown in Figure 8.4. Exploring that figure, what do you think are the major issues for the clinic to consider?

IDENTIFY IMPROVEMENTS

When presenting the data to all the stakeholders it should be possible to identify any specific improvements in practice that are needed, since: 'there is no point in describing a health care problem if nothing is done to ameliorate it' (Crombie et al 1993). There are two steps to this: assessing or diagnosing the reasons for not meeting the standards and then deciding on the most effective way of attempting to tackle the problem. Time must be spent on this stage of the audit since it is, after all, the whole

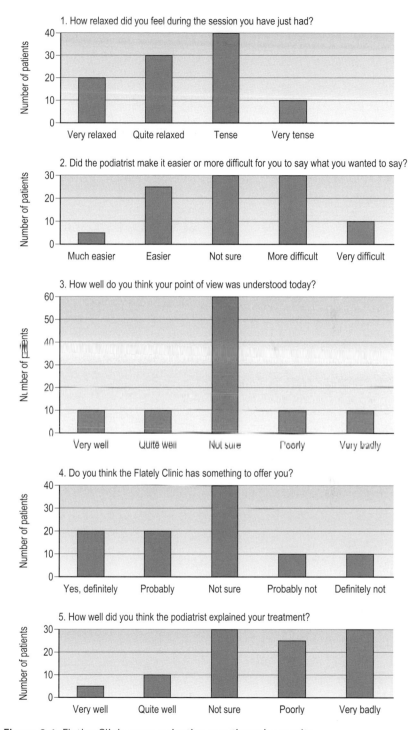

Figure 8.4 Flatley Clinic communication questionnaire results.

point of the audit! There are some key points that have to be considered at this stage:

- Prioritize short- and long-term targets
- Specify time limits
- Consider what sort of help is required (both internally and externally)
- What exactly has to change
- Potential barriers to change
- Most likely way of achieving change.

EXERCISE

The Flatley Clinic noted that, on the basis of the survey, patients did not feel the treatment was being clearly explained by the podiatrist. What sort of action do you think the clinic could introduce to improve this?

DEVELOPING ACTION PLANS

An action plan has to be produced which outlines what is to be done, who is to do it and what the time frame is to be. Finally, in order to complete the cycle, plans must be made for a re-audit at a specified date in the future. The changes required may be large or small – a minor change in practice or some educational input for the whole clinical team. Obviously such plans will require a different order of changes and consequent actions.

At the Flatley Clinic, communication with patients concerning their treatment was especially noted to be lacking. As a consequence, the

Table 8.5 Action plan

Problem identified	Suggested action	Staff responsible	Planned completion date	Actual date of completion
Communication with patients about treatment	Development of leaflets for common conditions detailing treatment	Head of Podiatry	April 2008	

action plan (Table 8.5) highlighted this as an issue. The suggestion was to develop a series of leaflets on common podiatric conditions and the treatment undertaken for these. The Head of Podiatry took responsibility for these developments, although he allocated different conditions to different podiatrists and relied on some freely available resources.

EXERCISE

Consider what other actions are required based on the audit. Complete the action plan sheet under the appropriate headings.

In some cases the audit may need to address wider concerns associated with the delivery of patient care. Therefore, the following may also need to be considered in order to complete the process:

- *Structure*: The premises, staffing, access to support services, diagnostic and treatment equipment
- *Processes*: Waiting times, patient recall, investigations, diagnosis, record keeping
- *Outcomes*: Therapy, improvements and adverse events.

IMPLEMENTATION

Somebody – usually the lead clinician – needs to take responsibility for implementing the action plan. This may, as in the Flatley Clinic, mean referring the action plan to others. However, it should be up to the responsible individual to develop a realistic action plan which takes into account factors outside the control of the group and to provide feedback to those involved in the audit, at least concerning any actions planned or taken. Ultimately, it is up to the responsible individual to confirm that audit findings have been acted upon and to provide reasons for lack of action where this has not been taken.

START AGAIN!

Remember: it is an audit cycle – at this stage you should also consider a date for re-audit and if no re-audit is to be carried out, the reasons why this is the case. Obviously, at the re-audit you can consider whether the improvements have been made – and if not, why not. Remember, the design, implementation and purpose of an audit are undermined if the monitoring of the implementation of recommendations from these activities is absent and the quality loop that underpins any quality activity is left incomplete (Berk et al 2003). A common difficulty which can lead to confusion between audit and research is that often only the first steps of the audit are completed. Hence, the audit will highlight the problems and the deficiencies of the process and the audit team will take this no further. This is not sufficient for an audit – although it may be for research. In research, once the study has been undertaken and some dissemination of the results has been completed, this may be considered the end of the process. It is not assumed that there will be any attempt to correct the deficiencies as a result of the research but this should be the case in audit. However, it could be expected that the research will generate evidence that may be used to inform future standards (Crombie et al 1993): 'The difference is between adding to the body of medical knowledge and ensuring that knowledge is effectively used.'

CONCLUSION

This chapter has outlined the reasons why audit may be undertaken and the process by which it is conducted. Furthermore, the key distinctions between audit and research activity were highlighted. If there is uncertainty as to whether the proposed investigation should be classified as audit or research, there is a simple question that can guide you: 'What is the overall purpose of the work?' If the remit is to improve care in a direct and specific way, and with an intention to return to the clinical area to monitor the situation in the future, then it should be considered an audit.

There are clear similarities and differences between audit and research. However, it should not be seen in this stark way: there are no clear boundaries and the interface between research and audit is important – they are nothing without one another. The audit cycle probably begins and ends with research (with research in the middle as well!) and the value of research can only be appreciated with a clear audit.

SUMMARY POINTS

- During the last two decades the context of healthcare has altered considerably and there is now a greater focus on evidence-based practice and clinical effectiveness.
- The audit process is a multi-professional activity and should not be confined to medicine or, indeed, to any mono-professional group.
- Sometimes there can be areas of uncertainty in which it may be problematic about deciding whether the investigation is research or audit.
- There can be a temptation to submit work as audit rather than research due to the difficulties in obtaining research approval – or rather the perception of difficulty.
- Discussion with other members of the clinical team may assist in the identification of the audit topic.
- Once the audit topic has been agreed with the audit team, it is essential to establish appropriate standards or criteria against which current practice can be assessed.
- A key step in the audit cycle is the assessment of practice against standards, and this may involve similar methods to those used in research.
- The data obtained through audit should be analysed using techniques akin to those employed in research.
- Data produced from the audit can be summarized by descriptive statistics and can be presented in summary through appropriate tables, figures and so on. However, it is essential that this presentation illustrates the extent to which the standard has, or has not, been met.
- The final step is in the discussion of the results with colleagues about the areas that need to be modified and improved.

DISCUSSION POINTS

1. Who should take the responsibility for clinical audit in your clinic? What is most likely to lead to improvements in patient care?
2. What are the similarities and differences between audit and research?
3. What research skills are required for audit?
4. Which of the following are involved in clinical governance and what is their role?:
   - Research and development
   - Evidence-based practice
   - Risk management
   - Financial management
   - Clinical audit.
5. What key areas in your podiatric practice do you think would benefit from audit? Outline how you would go about it.

REFERENCES

Baker 2002, Berk M, Callaly T, Hyland M 2003 The evolution of clinical audit as a tool for quality improvement. J Eval Clin Pract 9(2):251–257

Clinical Audit Central Office 2000 How to … Tell the difference between audit and research. United Bristol Healthcare Trust Clinical Audit Central Office, Bristol, p 1–3

Cooper J, Benjamin M 2004 Clinical audit in practice. Nursing Standard 18(28):47–53

Crombie IK, Davies HTO, Abraham SCS, Florey C 1993 The audit handbook. Wiley, Chichester

Department of Health 1989 Working for patients. DH, London

Department of Health 1993 Report of the taskforce on the strategy for research in nursing, midwifery and health visiting. DH, London

Department of Health 2001 Research Governance Framework for Health and Social Care. DH, London. Online. Available: www.dh.gov.uk/assetRoot/ 04/01/47/57/04014757.pdf

Department of Health 2005 How to apply ethics to clinical audit. DH, London Online. Available. www.ubht.nhs.uk/ClinicalAudit/docs/HowTo/ Ethics.pdf. See also: 'How to' guides. Online. Available: www.ubht.nhs.uk/ClinicalAudit/ HowTo.htm

DiMatteo MR 2004a Variations in patients' adherence to medical recommendations: a quantitative review of 50 years of research. Med Care 42(3):200–209

DiMatteo MR 2004b The role of effective communication with children and their families in fostering adherence to pediatric regimens. Patient Educ Couns 55(3):339–344

Jones AM, Bamford B 2004 The other face of research governance. BMJ 329(7460):280–281

Kneafsey R, Howarth M 2004 Research governance and the art of defence. Clin Effectiveness Nurs 8(2):66–67

National Institute for Health and Clinical Excellence 2002 Principles for best practice in clinical audit. NICE, London. Online. Available: www.nice.org.uk/page.aspx?o= 29058

Shakib S, Phillips PA 2003 The Australian Centre For Evidence-based Clinical Practice Generic Audit Tool: Auditmaker for health professionals. J Eval Clin Pract 9(2):259–263

Smith R 1992 Audit and research. BMJ 305:905–906

Smith R 2000 Babies and consent: yet another NHS scandal. But it should lead to improvements in research governance within the NHS. BMJ 320(7245):1285 1286

Stevenson FA, Cox S, Britten B, Dundar Y 2004 A systematic review of the research on communication between patients and health care professionals about medicines: the consequences for concordance. Health Expect 7(3):235–245

Trinder L, Reynolds S (eds) 2000 Evidence-based practice: a critical appraisal. Blackwell Science, Oxford

UBHT 2007 Clinical audit. United Bristol Healthcare NHS Trust, Bristol. Online. Available: www.ubht.nhs.uk/ClinicalAudit

Watson R, Manthorpe J 2002 Research governance: for whose benefit? J Adv Nurs 39(6):515–516

Chapter 9

Doing it at work

Be careful about reading health books. You may die of a misprint.

Mark Twain

LEARNING OUTCOMES

By the end of this chapter you will be able to:
- Understand the Research Governance Framework and how it can impact on your research process
- Comprehend the importance of developing a research protocol and monitoring the study and how it meets the original research plan
- Realize the importance of peer review of your research proposal
- Understand the need and requirements for ethical review of your research
- Appreciate the importance of informed consent and recognize the skills needed to develop patient information sheets
- Explore the data protection requirements associated with your research activity in the NHS.

INTRODUCTION

Attempting to complete research in the NHS is often viewed as a tiresome activity that gets in the way of clinical work, but the outcomes and support are well worth it! Indeed, it has to be remembered that research is the backbone to all our professional practice. This is recognized by the government, policy makers and managers and it is stressed that it should be central to our professional and service development. The Research Governance Framework (DH 2005, p. 2) states:

> The Government is committed to enhancing the contribution of research to health and social care. Research is essential to the successful promotion and protection of health and wellbeing, and also to modern, effective health and social care services. [...] Proper governance of research is essential to ensure that the public can have confidence in, and benefit from, quality research in health and social care. The public has a right to expect high scientific, ethical and financial standards, transparent decision-making processes, clear allocation of responsibilities and robust monitoring arrangements.

The Research Governance Framework was first introduced into healthcare in 2001 (and revised in 2005) and was established in response to the adverse publicity in Bristol[1] (child heart surgery), North Staffordshire[2] (children being entered into trials without their or their parent's consent) and Alder Hay[3] (retention of children's organs) that led to crises in the public's confidence in health research. The Framework sets out, clearly, to safeguard the rights and well being of *all participants* in health research, including investigators, organizations and patients themselves. Although the document appears unwieldy, prescriptive and overbearing, it simply boils down to formalizing good research practice that should always occur anyway.

CLINICAL TIP

Research should be central to our professional practice.

Case Study

Nicola is an experienced and committed podiatrist (unlike the one mentioned in Chapter 4), working for a local NHS Trust. Her main referrals are paediatrics with verruca that she treats with standard therapy. Nicola has been treating verrucae all her professional career and realizes that, without treatment, most will disappear after 6–12 months and leave no scar. This is particularly true in children and young adults. Sometimes they last longer but rarely more than 12–18 months. She appreciates that treatment can clear the warts quickly (or at least quicker than no treatment) but also acknowledges that it is time-consuming and can be painful. The first line of treatment, as recommended by the Cochrane Review (Gibbs et al 2003), suggested that the application of mild acid (e.g. salicylic acid, cantharidin, dichloroacetic acid) topically will help treat plantar warts. This treatment, which often requires multiple applications over the course of several weeks, disintegrates viral cells and allows healthy skin cells to replace them. However, it does take several weeks to complete and although speeding up the process this has to be balanced against the pain, discomfort and time involved which may be considered excessive given the outcomes obtained. The Cochrane Review rated the randomized controlled trials (RCTs) of local treatments for cutaneous warts as generally weak because of poor methodology and reporting. Additionally, the average cure rate for placebo preparations approached 30%. However, the conclusion to the Cochrane Review (Gibbs et al 2003, p. 1) was:

> The best available evidence was for simple topical treatments containing salicylic acid, which are clearly better than placebo. Data pooled from six placebo-controlled trials show a cure rate of 144/191 (75%) compared with 89/185 (48%) in controls.

Nicola's view is that simply waiting for the verruca to go is the best thing to do and wants her patients to realize this as well. However, her patients – or mainly the parents of her patients – actually want some form of treatment to happen. Nicola decides to investigate this further and comes up with two broad areas of research she wishes to investigate:

- Will a sham treatment incorporating saline solution rather than salicylic acid be just as effective as the first-line treatment?
- Will better information to her patients reduce the need for (as Nicola sees it) unnecessary treatment?

She decides that these are two areas she wants to study and sets about completing some research in her workplace to answer these questions. Before starting her research (and she is itching to get going) she contacts a podiatrist colleague from the university who has engaged in some research previously. He mentions the Research Governance Framework and urges her to fully consider the implications of the requirements for her research ambitions.

[1.] http://bmj.bmjjournals.com/cgi/content/full/323/7306/181
[2.] http://bmj.bmjjournals.com/cgi/content/full/320/7245/1285
[3.] http://www.pubmedcentral.nih.gov/articlerender.fcgi?artid = 1119515

EXERCISE

What are the research and ethical issues in the choice of Nicola's research questions?

SO WHAT IS THE RESEARCH GOVERNANCE FRAMEWORK?

Research Governance is a specific regulation framework that was issued by the Department of Health and covers all research that involves human subjects who have been recruited from either health or social care settings. It was initially implemented in 2001/2 and was updated in 2005. In essence, from April 2001, all research involving patients, human samples, patient data or NHS staff or facilities *has* to meet the specific requirements set out in the Framework.

WHY WAS THE FRAMEWORK INTRODUCED?

The Framework was introduced in response to a series of scandals emanating from research in the NHS (as discussed above). The aim of the Framework was an attempt at restoring public confidence in research. The essence of the Framework is to provide a system that safeguards all of those that participate in research. The Framework addresses the needs of universities and health and social care organizations to work closely together to manage research quality and safeguard patients. Furthermore, researchers would be supported to conduct high-quality research which would protect both themselves and the participants in the research.

HOW WILL THE FRAMEWORK AFFECT YOU?

Everyone who conducts research in the health or social services will be expected to adhere to the Framework, so if you intend to conduct any research it will impact on you! The main requirements are outlined in Table 9.1.

Hopefully, for the most part, the Framework merely formalizes good research practice that is already in place in day-to-day research activities.

However, before you start, key questions that you should ask yourself are: 'Has this project been done before?' and 'Do I have the capability to do this project?' In previous chapters we spoke about formulating a research question and then searching the literature about the topic. Returning to our case study, Nicola did a quick review of the literature (following the advice in Chapter 4) and found several studies including the Cochrane Review of verruca treatment (Gibbs et al 2003). In light of these studies, the comprehensive review and the recognition that she did

Table 9.1 Requirements of the Research Governance Framework

Requirement	Impact
Research projects have to be formally approved before they can begin	It is no good deciding on Monday that you want to do some research and start on Tuesday
Approval procedures should take account of the scientific quality of the project and the capacity and experience of the researcher(s) to complete the research	It is not enough to have a simple 'research idea'; there is a need for it to be investigated fully and to be scientifically robust. The research team must also have the capacity (in terms of skills and time) to undertake the research
All research must have appropriate ethics approval before the study can start	There are different processes dependent on which area of the health service you are in (see later for more details). However, whatever your organization and your study design, you will need ethical approval *before* the study starts
Research involving patients must have the approval of the appropriate care organization before the study can commence	Written approval from your care organization must be obtained *before* you start
There must be clear procedures to secure informed consent from participants and systems to check that this happens consistently	Informed consent means that participants need information about the study and a protocol needs to be developed in order to provide this information
The research must be actively monitored to ensure that it is conducted in accordance with the protocol	A system must be in place to check that the study is being carried out properly throughout the study period
Legal requirements such as health and safety and data protection must be complied with	As it says on the tin!

CLINICAL TIP

Before starting any research, always do a thorough literature review and reflect on your own capabilities.

not have at her disposal the resources (time, money, equipment and so on) to perform a large scale RCT that would satisfactorily add to the literature, she decided not to progress her first research question (quality of the traditional treatment) any further. However, she was still keen to explore the value of information leaflets on the choice of verruca treatment. As her literature review had found limited evidence or even research studies on this topic, she felt that this was an area worthy of further investigation. She therefore set out to develop a research protocol in this area that was within the context of the Research Governance Framework.

The Research Governance Framework is based on seven core principles which are worth exploring in more detail here.

1. RESEARCH PROJECTS HAVE TO BE FORMALLY APPROVED BEFORE THEY CAN BEGIN

The Research Governance Framework requires all health/social care research to be peer reviewed. There are already many systems in place for externally funded projects to be reviewed and it is likely that such a system (or panel) exists within your organization. Obviously, it may not be in the local clinic but may be at the Trust, PCT or other central health or social care organizational level. If your research proposal has to go through an ethics committee (and it is probable that it will) then most research ethics committees will expect principal investigators (PIs) to provide evidence of peer review. Usually (although not always) applications can be submitted straight to the ethics panel if they:

- are externally funded
- can demonstrate evidence of independent external review specific to the proposed project
- have the appropriate R&D approval signatures.

However, a copy of the independent review will need to be attached to the ethics panel submission.

When an independent review is undertaken the expert reviewers will ask themselves a series of questions (sometimes these will be formally listed, and sometimes not). In order to best prepare yourself for the review, and as a matter of good practice, you should ask yourself the following questions about your research:

- Is the research question important? This is in terms of both:
  - the particular field of research as a whole
  - the value of the research for health or social care.
- Is the background information provided relevant and of good quality?
- What are the strengths and weaknesses of the design and the methods of the proposed plan of investigation?
- Does the research presents ethical concerns? If so, does the plan of investigation address these concerns?
- Is the analysis suggested (whether this be statistical or qualitative) appropriate?
- Does the research team have the capacity and expertise to complete the proposed study?
- Have the resource requirements been adequately stated and are they available?

KEY CONCEPT

REMEMBER 'I SWEAT'

I : Importance and relevance?
S : Strengths?
W : Weaknesses?
E : Ethics?
A : Analysis?
T : Team and resources?

CLINICAL TIP

The Research Governance Framework merely formalizes good practice.

As emphasized throughout this chapter, most of the Research Governance Framework is about good practice. Any researcher worth their salt should be asking themselves these questions anyway – the Framework merely formalizes these in order to protect all involved in the research process.

Back to our intrepid podiatric researcher and the review of her project. Given her commitment to her research she had already organized a peer evaluation from her local Trust and had also discussed it with colleagues at a continuing professional development event. On the basis of the feedback she received, she developed the project further by:

- introducing a qualitative element to the research to obtain rich data and on the basis of this would develop a questionnaire for a larger scale study
- completing a thorough ethical analysis prior to submitting the proposal to the Ethics Committee
- completing a thorough cost analysis of the project – what resources were required and how much it would cost to complete, both in terms of financial costs and the researcher's time and administrative support required
- appreciating that she did not have sufficient research experience, other than some undergraduate and postgraduate projects. In order to improve this position, she teamed up with colleagues from a local university.

2. APPROVAL PROCEDURES SHOULD TAKE ACCOUNT OF THE SCIENTIFIC QUALITY OF THE PROJECT AND THE CAPACITY AND EXPERIENCE OF THE RESEARCHER(S) TO COMPLETE THE RESEARCH

As we can see from the above approval process, there is a need to ensure that the quality of both the researcher(s) and the project is sufficient in order to complete the research. This may not only be about the quality of the individual researcher but also about the quality of the research team. An individual researcher may be inexperienced in research, the topic area or specific research skills or elements of any of these. However, it is unlikely that a team will lack all of the essential skills. Therefore, if you are new to research, or feel that you do not have the capacity to complete the research, then consider teaming up with colleagues. Indeed, team research is often a more positive and constructive experience than working alone.

The organization itself should have the research capacity to support and develop new researchers. Indeed, the Research Governance Framework (DH 2005) suggests that:

CLINICAL TIP

Remember to team up with experienced local researchers to develop your idea and your skills further.

The organization plays its role in developing research capacity with appropriate training and updating. This includes taking action to ensure that the diversity of the workforce reflects society, and developing the capacity of consumers to participate.

3. ALL RESEARCH MUST HAVE APPROPRIATE ETHICS APPROVAL BEFORE THE STUDY CAN START

There are a number of ethics committees associated with conducting research in the NHS at present – although the number and nature of these changes regularly. The National Research Ethics Service (NRES – http://www.nres.npsa.nhs.uk/) is the over-arching body across the UK. NRES replaced COREC (**Central Office for Research Ethics Committee**) from the 1st April 2007. NRES comprises both the central function which was formerly undertaken by COREC and the NHS Research Ethics Committees (RECs) in England. The NRES provides the following services:

- Ethical guidance to local Research Ethics Committees.
- A quality assurance framework for the ethics committees.

- A UK-wide framework for ethical service.
- Steamlining of the ethical and regulatory processes.

NRES in England works closely with colleagues with similar responsibilities in Scotland, Wales and Northern Ireland (OREC: Office for Research Ethics Committees). The web site provided by NRES (see p. 150) provides up-to-date and comprehensive information on the Research Ethics Committee system in the United Kingdom. It helpfully provides information for patients/the public, applications and for those working with RECs. It also lists the most recent updates to the guidance and the application forms.

An application to a REC is required for any research proposal involving (taken from the Governance Arrangement for NHS Research Ethics Committees, 2001):

a. patients and users of the NHS. This includes all potential research participants recruited by virtue of the patient or user's past or present treatment by, or use of, the NHS. It includes NHS patients treated under contracts with private sector institutions
b. individuals identified as potential research participants because of their status as relatives or carers of patients and users of the NHS, as defined above
c. access to data, organs or other bodily material of past and present NHS patients
d. fetal material and IVF involving NHS patients
e. the recently dead in NHS premises
f. the use of, or potential access to, NHS premises or facilities
g. NHS staff – recruited as research participants by virtue of their professional role.

An additional warning at this state: the application form to REC attempts to cover all of these potential eventualities and hence is exceedingly long and convoluted (the form can be obtained from http://www.nres.npsa.nhs.uk/applicants/index.htm). Because of this people are often put off by the extreme length of the application form. However, many of the questions are not relevant to all studies and can simply be ignored. So even though the application can look daunting and you may be worried about the length of the form you should not let this put you off – most of the questions may not be relevant.

CLINICAL TIP

Don't be put off by the length of the ethics application form.

Things to think about when making an ethics application

The emphasis throughout this chapter has been about the Framework merely being a reflection of good practice but formalizing this more fully. It is the same with the ethics form – you should address all of the questions on the application form but this should be relatively easy if you have planned and developed the study appropriately. In order to assist with this process, below are some questions for you to consider before making an ethics application.

Scientific design and conduct of study

1. Is this research worthwhile and will it answer the question the researcher has posed?
2. Is there assessment of the risks/benefits for research participants?

3. How appropriate is the study design in relation to the objectives of the study?
4. What statistical methodology will be employed (including sample size calculation)? What is the potential for reaching a sound conclusion with the smallest number of research participants?
5. Does the research involve a placebo? How ethical is this? Will subjects be told?
6. Are subjects blinded to the study arms? (i.e. are they unaware which treatment they will be receiving?)
7. How have the predictable risks and inconveniences been justified in relation to the anticipated benefits for research participants, other present and future patients, concerned communities and the wider public?
8. If control arms are being proposed, how has their use been justified?
9. What are the criteria for prematurely withdrawing research participants?
10. What are the criteria for suspending or terminating the research study as a whole?
11. What provisions have been made for monitoring and assessing the conduct of the research?
12. Does the research site meet the study requirements, in terms of supporting staff, available facilities and emergency procedures?
13. How will the results of the research be reported and published?
14. Are systems in place to monitor all aspects of the quality of the research?
15. Is all research information recorded, handled and stored in a way that allows accurate reporting, interpretation and verification?
16. Is the available non-clinical and clinical information on an investigational medical product adequate to support the proposed clinical research?
17. Are there any circumstances that might lead to conflicts of interest that may affect the independent judgement of the researcher(s)?

Recruitment of research participants

1. How will initial contact and recruitment be conducted?
2. How will information be conveyed to potential research participants or their representatives?
3. What are the inclusion criteria for research participants, and are they justified?
4. What are the exclusion criteria for research participants, and are they justified?

Care and protection of research participants

1. How safe is the intervention to be used in the proposed research?
2. Are there any plans to withdraw or withhold standard therapies or clinical management protocols for the purpose of the research? If so, how has such action been justified?
3. What steps will be taken if research participants withdraw?
4. What arrangements have been made for informing participants' GPs of their participation in the research?

5. If applicable, will the study product be made available to the research participants following the research?
6. Will the research participants incur any financial costs as a result of their participation in the research?
7. Will the research participants receive any rewards/compensation for their participation in the study?
8. What are the insurance and indemnity arrangements? Has provision for compensation/treatment been made in proportion to the risk?
9. Are there monitoring and reporting arrangements of risks in place?
10. Is the right to physical and mental integrity and privacy and protection safeguarded?
11. Are medical care and medical decisions the responsibility of an appropriately qualified doctor?

Protection of research participants' confidentiality

1. Who will have access to the personal data of the research participants, including medical records and biological samples, with justification?
2. How will consent for the acquisition of personal data/samples be obtained?
3. What measures have been taken to ensure the confidentiality and security of personal information concerning research participants?
4. To what extent will personal information about participants be anonymous?
5. How long will the data/samples be kept?
6. How will they be stored?
7. To which other countries, if any, will the data samples be sent? Will data in particular be sent outside the EU? (There are less stringent data protection laws in some countries.)

Consent

1. How will consent be obtained?
2. Is the information given appropriate, complete and understandable?
3. What is the justification for including in the research individuals who cannot consent? What arrangements have been made for obtaining consent of such individuals?
4. Where research subjects are unable to write, has provision been made for consent to be obtained orally with at least one witness?

Community considerations

1. Will there be impact on the local community?
2. What steps have been taken to consult with the concerned communities during the course of the study design process?
3. In what manner will the results of the research be made available to the research participants and concerned communities?

Suitability of the researcher

1. The researcher's CV (and supervision of student if applicable).
2. Any conflicts of interest.
3. Payments to researchers.
4. That individuals conducting the research are appropriately trained, educated and experienced or appropriately supervised.

Research involving children

When reviewing research involving children, here are some useful questions taken from the Guidelines from the Royal College of Paediatrics and Child Health (2000) and Edwards and McNamee (2005):

1. Appropriate consent procedures must be in place from either the child or parents, depending on the child's competence.
2. The applicant should confirm that the research results cannot be obtained from any other group of research subjects.
3. The protocol should ensure that the consent obtained represents the child's presumed will and can be evoked at any time without detriment to the child.
4. The protocol should ensure the child receives information on risks and benefits according to their capacity to understand from staff experienced with children.
5. The protocol should ensure that the explicit wish of the child to refuse to participate or withdraw at any time is considered and acted upon by the investigator or, where appropriate, the principal investigator.
6. The protocol and patient information sheet should make clear that no incentives or inducements are given apart from reasonable travel and out of pocket expenses where warranted.
7. The research design/protocol/patient information sheet should address the need to minimize pain, discomfort and fear and other foreseeable risks. There should be provision to monitor and report on any of these issues.

There are also various questions that you should ask yourself when considering research into genetics, fetal material or radioactivity (including X-rays) but these are not replicated here.

EXERCISE

Consider the research project mentioned in the case study. What sort of ethical considerations are apparent?

Despite the guidance available on various websites and from the REC, there are still a number of common problems that can occur. For example:

Statistical information

- Statistical advice should be sought.
- Sample size should be justified on scientific grounds.

Patient information sheet

- Use the standard format available on the COREC website.
- Use plain English which can be easily understood by participants.
- Separate from consent form.
- On locally headed paper.
- Include date and version number.

Consent

CLINICAL TIP

Ethics must be central to
your research process.

**Those whose first
language is not English**

4. RESEARCH
INVOLVING PATIENTS
MUST HAVE THE
APPROVAL OF THE
APPROPRIATE CARE
ORGANIZATION
BEFORE THE STUDY
CAN COMMENCE

5. THERE MUST BE
CLEAR PROCEDURES
TO SECURE INFORMED
CONSENT FROM
PARTICIPANTS AND
SYSTEMS TO CHECK
THAT THIS HAPPENS
CONSISTENTLY

- Use the standard format available on the COREC website
- Separate from information sheet.
- On locally headed paper.
- Signed and dated by the participant and the person who obtains consent.
- Obtained by someone experienced/trained in obtaining consent.
- Include date and version number.

- The exclusion of those whose first language is not English should be justified. Note that such people may speak and understand English perfectly well.

You must ensure that the appropriate care organization – your hospital Trust, your PCT or your healthcare facility – has given you written approval for the study and this must be within clear guidelines. This is not simply a matter of getting a nod of approval in the corridor or the refectory: you must ensure that you have express written permission to do the research. There are usually scientific scrutiny committees and/or research governance committees that can provide approval. There is a standard form for applying for permission to undertake research in the NHS and this can be found on the web at www.nresform.org.uk. (The national NHS R&D application form has now been merged with Part C of the national REC application form to create an integrated Site-Specific Information Form (SSIF). The new form can be used to apply both for site-specific assessment and R&D approval at NHS sites, except in Northern Ireland, where separate arrangements will be in place for R&D applications. You should check this website frequently because the forms and guidance are updated regularly.)

Informed consent must be obtained from human participants involved in research. Therefore, people who are asked to participate in medical research must be able to make a sensible decision. In order to do this, they must have sufficient information about the project. In this way, they should be able to make a free and informed decision about their participation. This is relatively easy for adults but if the research involves children or vulnerable adults then there are different responsibilities for the researcher. For example, with children, parents have the ethical and legal responsibility for giving consent on behalf of their child. Even though this is the case, the information has to be provided for both children and adults. This may mean that distinct, separate information sheets are provided so that the child's right to be informed is not infringed.

Under research governance regulations, researchers must provide participants with good quality, understandable information sheets. The information provided to participants and their families must be sufficient to enable legally valid consent to be obtained. The information that has to be provided should be devised and presented in a manner suitable for the recipient – whether this be a child, an adult or perhaps a vulnerable adult group.

Writing your information sheet

The information given to patients must be easy for the general public to understand. Although it should be brief, it must be inclusive of all relevant facts and pertinent information and should be presented and written in an informative style. It is important that the style is appropriate – not patronizing or coercive, but straightforward and informative. It should be written in a simplistic style – sentences should be short and jargon-free, and medical terminology must be avoided or explained (see the Glossary at the end of this book for some examples and how common research terms such as 'placebo' or 'controlled trial' can be explained in lay terminology). The writer of the information sheet should ensure that the reading age of information sheets is approximately 12 years, in line with most public information documents in the UK.

KEY CONCEPT

Readability is of key importance when producing information sheets. It can be easy to check the reading age of the material you use, using the Microsoft Word spell check. At the end of a spell check, a list of characteristics of the document is presented. You should aim for a Flesch–Kincaid Grade Level of 7–8. This corresponds to an age of 12–13. Other word processing packages will have similar features.

Information to include in your information sheet

Your proposed research should be described fully and some of the following points should be taken into account:

1. *Title*: This should be self-explanatory to a lay person.
2. *Invitation paragraph*: You should explain that the patient is being asked to take part in a research project.
3. *The aim of the project*: Again this should be presented in simplistic lay terms.
4. *Why is the project being done?*: It may be clear to you, but you have to explain why to the participant and to colleagues and peers.
5. *How is the project to be done?*:
   - Explain exactly what will be done to the patient, i.e. what will happen to them?
   - Explain which parts of the project are additional to normal treatment:
     - When?
     - Where?
     - By whom?
     - How often?
   - Give details – this is what most people want to know. Include logistical details, e.g. transport arrangements, reimbursements, how long visits/procedures will last, etc.
   - Detail any lifestyle restrictions – for example, are there any dietary restrictions?
   - Some drug studies require pregnancy tests, or some form of declaration that contraception will be used. You will need to indicate this on the information sheets if it applies to your project.

6. *Are there risks and discomforts?*: State these carefully, and be honest. If you do not inform participants of risks that might influence their decision to participate in a project, you may be liable in law in the event of an untoward incident. Remember that risks and harms may include psychological or emotional factors, e.g. due to an intrusive questionnaire.
7. *What are the potential benefits?*: List the potential benefits to the subject and to others. Where there is likely to be no direct benefit to the participant, you should clearly state this. Where it is unknown how effective a new treatment will be, this must be clearly stated.
8. *What other treatments are available?*: What options are available if people choose not to participate in this project?
9. *What if new information becomes available?*: If new information becomes available during the course of the research you will need to tell the patient about this.
10. *What happens when the research stops?*: If the treatment will not be available after the research finishes, you should explain this to the patient. You should also explain what treatment will be available instead.
11. *Who will have access to the case/research records?*: In the case of a company-sponsored project, this will usually be the company producing the drug/device and a representative of the Research Ethics Committee. Who else will have access to the information and the records? Are they associated with your unit, or a local collaborator?
12. *What are the arrangements for compensation, should any harm come to the participant?*
13. *Do I have to take part in this project?*: Always include the following statement: 'If you decide, now or at a later stage, that you do not wish to participate in this research project, that is entirely your right, and will not in any way prejudice any present or future treatment.'
14. *Who is organizing and funding the project?*: For example, is it a pharmaceutical company, a charity or an academic institution?
15. *Who do I speak to if problems arise?*: Highlight the person to whom the participant should speak and how they can complain if they need to do so.
16. *Researcher with whom to have contact*: The name and contact details of the researcher and PI should be provided.

CLINICAL TIP

An information sheet must be clear and understandable.

6. THE RESEARCH MUST BE ACTIVELY MONITORED TO ENSURE THAT IT IS CONDUCTED IN ACCORDANCE WITH THE PROTOCOL

The research process must be monitored to ensure it matches that which was outlined in the original protocol. Ethical approval is normally for a 3-year period and an extension can be obtained only after writing to the Committee to explain the reasoning behind the protocol changes and/or extensions. Protocol amendments should be submitted to the REC by the lead investigator for re-appraisal if there are any changes to the original methodology (e.g. sample size, tests to be administered).

7. LEGAL REQUIREMENTS SUCH AS HEALTH AND SAFETY AND DATA PROTECTION MUST BE COMPLIED WITH

All legal requirements have to be complied with – this should be relatively obvious. However, the one area that raises issues for discussion is the Data Protection Act (1998). This Act has various elements:

1. Personal data shall be processed fairly and lawfully.
2. Personal data shall be obtained only for one or more specified and lawful purposes, and shall not be further processed in any manner incompatible with that purpose or those purposes.
3. Personal data shall be adequate, relevant and not excessive in relation to the purpose or purposes for which they are processed.
4. Personal data shall be accurate and, where necessary, kept up to date.
5. Personal data processed for any purpose or purposes shall not be kept for longer than is necessary for that purpose or those purposes.
6. Personal data shall be processed in accordance with the rights of data subjects under this Act.
7. Appropriate technical and organizational measures shall be taken against unauthorized or unlawful processing of personal data and against accidental loss or destruction of, or damage to, personal data.
8. Personal data shall not be transferred to a country or territory outside the European Economic Area unless that country or territory ensures an adequate level of protection for the rights and freedoms of data subjects in relation to the processing of personal data.

Overall points to remember

- The Act only concerns the personal data of living individuals. The data may be in manual (paper) or electronic format and include images (any means by which an individual is identified).
- Don't cause substantial distress or damage to the individuals whose data have been seen, used or held. Don't use the material to make or support decisions or measures that will affect data subjects.
- Keep any personal information held secure (protect from unauthorized access or transfer).
- Anonymizing names/personal details is good practice and the safest way to avoid an infringement of the Act. Anonymize as early as possible in the use of the data.
- Sensitivity generally diminishes over time.
- The researcher is liable for the personal data they take away and the subsequent use they make of such data.

Further guidance on the Data Protection Act (1998) can be found at www.informationcommissioner.gov.uk.

CONCLUSION

Research within the NHS is essential to the development of the service and to provide fully evidence-based practice. It is not simply about waiting for research to be published and disseminated – we should all be involved in the conduct and publication of research. This is not only about continuing professional development, but also about maximizing evidence-based service to our patients and clients. A series of unfortunate events in the 1990s/2000s led to the introduction of the Research Governance Framework that codified good research practice in the NHS. These elements should be central to the conduct of research within the health service: projects should be formally approved and of high scientific quality, with ethics at the centre of the project and clear allocation of responsibilities for everybody involved. The Framework assures all involved that the research is being completed to the highest possible standards.

SUMMARY POINTS

- Research is essential to the promotion and protection of health and well-being.
- The Research Governance Framework was introduced in 2001 with revisions in 2005 in response to a series of public health research scandals.
- All research involving NHS staff, facilities or patients has to meet the specific Framework requirements.
- All research has to be formally approved before commencement.
- All research should be peer reviewed for scientific quality and researcher capacity.
- All research must have ethical approval before it starts.
- Clear procedures to obtain informed consent from all participants must be part of the research process.
- All legal requirements must be complied with.
- The requirements of the Data Protection Act must be adhered to.
- Remember to provide information in a clear and concise fashion and minimize jargon.

DISCUSSION POINTS

1. What promoted the development of the Research Governance Framework?
2. What are the main principles of the Research Governance Framework?
3. What are the principal ethical considerations that have to be addressed when designing a research study?
4. Describe the following terms in lay language appropriate for a patient information sheet: 'Intervention study', 'Experimental design', 'Placebo controlled trial' and 'Qualitative data-set'.
5. What should you do with the data you collect from your research? How does the Data Protection Act influence your data collection and collation?

REFERENCES

Department of Health 2001 Governance arrangements for NHS Research Ethics Committees. DH, London

Department of Health 2005 Research Governance Framework for health and social care, 2nd edn. DH, London

Edwards SD, McNamee MJ 2005 Ethical concerns regarding guidelines for the conduct of clinical research on children. J Med Ethics 31:351–354

Gibbs S, Harvey I, Sterling JC, Stark R 2003 Local treatments for cutaneous warts (Cochrane Review). Cochrane Database Syst Rev (3):CD001781

Guidelines from the Royal College of Paediatrics and Child Health 2000 Arch Dis Child 82:177–182

Chapter 10

What it was all about

Now this is not the end. It is not even the beginning of the end. But it is, perhaps, the end of the beginning.

Winston Churchill

After presenting what may seem like a torrent of information, it is useful to take some time to consider just exactly what this was all about and answer the question: 'What was the point?' There is a strong temptation to tackle these issues at length, but we believe that there is a clear and simple rationale underpinning the entire text that can be summarized in a series of factual statements that do not require further extended discussion. Moreover, the key skills that were presented in the individual chapters can also be summarized in this way. Therefore, what is presented here is firstly a clear exposition of the background to the text, reminding us of exactly why we should devote some of our time to it, followed by a similarly clear exposition of the core skills that we must develop if we are to adopt an evidence-based approach to our practice.

WHY WE SHOULD TAKE EVIDENCE-BASED PRACTICE (EBP) SERIOUSLY

- EBP is an approach to clinical practice where the best available information is sought to ensure that each patient receives optimal care.
- EBP seems to be here to stay. The approach has been adopted by governments, who see it as an important mechanism for establishing and ensuring quality healthcare, and for ensuring they secure the 'best bang for their buck'.
- Any doubt as to the influence of EBP can be dispelled by considering its influence on strategy and policy development in the NHS (DH 2000, 2003, NHSE 1997) and in the prominence and authority of organizations such as the National Institute for Health and Clinical Excellence.
- Whilst there is a clear political dimension to EBP, an important factor attracting individuals to the health professions is a desire to care for

people and improve their quality of life. Therefore, a vital dimension to EBP is the opportunity it offers health professionals to realize this original aspiration – to be involved in the provision of quality care to patients. This is perhaps the strongest motivation for adopting the principles of EBP, irrespective of any political influence.

- There is evidence that allied health professionals have adopted these principles and recognize their value in developing an excellent, patient-centred service (Upton & Upton 2006).

- However, the development of a suitable evidence base upon which to build practice is dependent on the development of a critical mass of healthcare professionals who are either in a position to conduct research or to implement scientific findings (Hicks & Hennessey 1997, Rafferty et al 2003).

- EBP focuses on the clinical implementation of scientific findings. Therefore, the development of this critical mass of healthcare professionals is dependent on the individual members of that profession learning and practising EBP.

- EBP, therefore, will only succeed if 'coal face' health professionals develop the necessary skills. These 'coal face' professionals could be termed 'research consumers' and EBP is essentially a process that creates more discerning research consumers.

- It is entirely feasible that, if individual professions fail to develop an appropriate evidence base, funding will diminish as those professions which do develop an appropriate evidence base are (justifiably) prioritized to receive funds.

We believe that these facts are a reality, are inescapable and justify us spending time learning about the process.

THE CRITICAL SKILLS NEEDED TO PRACTISE EBP

- EBP is a system of approaching clinical practice where evidence is sought regarding the care of individual patients.

- There are five steps to the process, each of which was addressed in an individual chapter.

- Step 1 (Chapter 2) involves formulating a good question: it is inappropriate to simply ask: 'What is the best way of treating this condition?' We must seek information concerning the best way of treating this particular expression of this particular pathology, in this particular patient and in terms of the required outcome.

- Step 2 (Chapter 4) involves conducting an efficient literature search to provide the information required to answer our question. The literature base is vast and, as such, only a well-planned and carefully executed search will yield the best information that exists.

- Step 3 (Chapter 5) involves critical evaluation of the literature found in the literature search to determine its quality and suitability for informing practice. This is essentially a quality appraisal, which we can conduct using critical appraisal tools as a guide. These tools are comprised of a series of questions concerning important aspects of the study.

- Critical appraisal can proceed using appraisal tools, but more detailed appraisal requires an understanding of the central issues involved in research design (Chapter 6).
- Critical appraisal is conducted with the ultimate aim of changing clinical practice. We must think carefully, balancing the available evidence, before changing our practice, and where we do choose to change our practice, we must do so in a systematic, controlled manner so that we can understand the effects associated with any changes (Chapter 7).
- The topic of audit should be considered an essential part of the process of EBP, as it provides the mechanism for developing an understanding of our effectiveness (Chapter 8).

NOW THIS IS NOT THE END...GETTING MOTIVATED!

The quote at the start of this chapter is entirely appropriate and is worth exploring briefly. Learning about the skills associated with EBP is not a dry academic exercise. It represents the first steps in adopting an approach to practice which promises, amongst other things, increased clinical effectiveness, increased professional respect associated with the ability to provide quality care, and increased job satisfaction. Each healthcare professional surely wants to offer their patients the very best care available. Berwick (1998), in an excellent (and highly recommended) article based on his speech at the 50th anniversary of the NHS conference, presented the principles he considered to be prerequisites for the development of a benchmark NHS. This excellent discourse presented many important points, but two seem particularly relevant in concluding this text. First is the sentiment conveyed in the quote, 'If only we knew what we knew, we would be geniuses.' This is how EBP should be considered – it is a process that shows us how to make sense of the vast healthcare literature, drawing out good-quality information concerning patient care. Secondly, it was asserted that, 'Improvement comes from knowledge.' The rationale for this was illustrated superbly in a quotation taken from the inaugural speech by the president of the Royal College of Physicians in 2001:

> If we know that someone – anyone – in the NHS has achieved a level of care or outcome that outdistances the rest of us, we have not just an opportunity, but a sacred duty, to put that example to use everywhere as our new standard of practice, or go one better. Let physicians never confuse professionalism with insularity. The NHS is our close and welcome partner in finding, documenting, and helping us to learn from the best among us.

Although this quote refers to the NHS and physicians, the concepts are clearly relevant to all healthcare professionals. Adopting the principles of

EBP offers an excellent opportunity to 'raise our game', which, in addition to helping patients, can help us consolidate and develop our professional position. The gauntlet has been thrown down to all healthcare professions and each and every one of us must respond.

REFERENCES

Derwick DM 1998 Looking forward: the NHS: feeling well and thriving at 75. BMJ 317:57–61

Department of Health 2000 Meeting the challenge: strategy for the allied health professions. DH, London

Department of Health 2003 The StLaR HR Project – phase one consultation report. September–December 2003. DH, London

Hicks C, Hennessy D 1997 Mixed messages in nursing research: their contribution to the persisting hiatus between evidence and practice. J Adv Nursing 25:595–601

NHSE 1997 Research and development in primary care: National Working Group Report (The Mant Report). NHSE, Leeds

Rafferty AM, Traynor M, Thompson DR, Ilott I, White E 2003 Research in nursing, midwifery, and the allied health professions: a quantum leap required for quality research. BMJ 326:833–834

Upton D, Upton P 2006 Knowledge and use of evidence based practice by allied health and health science professionals. J Allied Health 35(3):127–133

Glossary of terms

AUDIT

(1) Defined by the Department of Health as: 'The systematic critical analysis of the quality of medical care, including the procedures used for diagnosis and treatment, the use of resources and the resulting outcome and quality of life for the patient.' (2) A process whereby an existing practice is evaluated to determine the extent to which it conforms to an established standard. The established standard can come from practice guidelines or from the consensus of stakeholders.

BIAS

A variable which acts to distort the outcome of a study. Sources of bias must be thoroughly considered when designing or appraising a study to ensure that the outcome occurred due to recognized factors and not because of another, biasing, influence. Can be thought of as a prejudice, or preference for one particular response.

BLINDING (in an RCT)

A desirable feature of a randomized controlled trial which increases its quality. A study can either be *single blind* or *double blind.* A single-blind study does not tell participants which treatment they are receiving so that this knowledge cannot influence their response. A double-blind study does not tell investigators which treatment the participants are receiving either, so that this knowledge cannot influence the information they record.

BOOLEAN OPERATORS

Logical ways of combining search strategies such as AND, OR and NOT.

CASE–CONTROL STUDY

A study design that can provide insight into the cause of a disease. A group of cases – who suffer from the disease of interest – are recruited and compared to a group of controls – who do not have the disease but are 'matched' to the cases. 'Matching' ensures that cases and controls are similar in as many important ways as possible. Differences between the groups may account for the development of the disease, and therefore may warrant further investigation. Case-control studies cannot prove *cause* – they can only identify that a variable is *associated* with a disease.

CASE SERIES

A case series represents an improvement over a case study because it describes not just one case, but a sequence. Provides slightly more convincing information than a case study, but is still a weak source of information. This is because we may be focusing on an unusual effect.

CASE STUDY

A description of a single case encountered, performed to highlight an interesting or unusual aspect of the case that can provide a learning experience for readers. Case studies provide weak evidence of a general effect because they may be describing the exception rather than the rule.

CATEGORICAL VARIABLE

A variable which falls into distinct groups which are mutually exclusive and cannot be hierarchically organized. An example is vegetables, where it is possible to categorize them in various ways. However, it is not possible, in any objective way, to say that one is better or bigger than another.

CAUSE/CAUSAL VARIABLE OR FACTOR

A causal relationship exists when a factor leads to a disease. Factors can also be associated, but that does not mean that they are causally related.

CHANCE

In any research study there is always the possibility – no matter how remote – that the results occurred purely by chance, i.e. because of some random, unexpected effect.

CLINICAL EFFECTIVENESS

Defined by the NHS Executive as: 'The extent to which specific clinical interventions, when deployed in the field for a particular patient or population, do what they are intended to do, i.e. maintain and improve health and secure the greatest possible health gain from available resources.'

CLINICAL GOVERNANCE

Defined by the Department of Health as: 'A framework through which NHS organizations are accountable for continuously improving the quality of their services and safeguarding high standards of care, by creating an environment in which excellence in clinical care will flourish.' The definition includes three key factors: recognizably high standards of care, transparent responsibility and accountability, and constant improvement.

COCHRANE COLLABORATION

The Cochrane Collaboration is an international group devoted to doing systematic reviews of the literature to answer common clinical problems. Divided into over 40 groups, each tackles a different perspective or organsystem. For example, the Stroke Working Group has done over 40 meta-analyses on important topics such as the use of thrombolytics, heparin and aspirin in acute stroke.

COHORT STUDY

Involves following a group of subjects over time. Information is gathered as the study proceeds and, as subjects develop health effects, it is possible to examine whether the variables on which information was gathered are responsible for these effects. A famous cohort study was the Framingham study of cardiovascular risk factors.

CONFIDENCE INTERVAL (CI)

A measure of the precision of a 'point estimate' – the average. It is defined technically as the range into which 95% of the observations fall. For example, if we record the age of a group of people, we can calculate the average. Calculating the 95% CI will tell us the range into which 95% of the samples ages fall. If it is narrow, the group is clustered around the mean; if it is broad, the group has a widely varying age. Any CI can be calculated, and sometimes 90 or 99% CIs are used.

CONFOUNDING FACTOR

A variable that acts to distort the outcome of a study.

CONSORT STATEMENT

A guideline setting out a series of standards that should be met by randomized controlled trials to maximize validity. CONSORT = **Con**solidated **S**tandards for **R**eporting **T**rials. A study satisfying more standards is deemed to be of a better quality, and therefore the results can be taken as more accurate, than a study satisfying fewer standards.

CONSTRUCT VALIDITY

The extent to which the test may be said to measure a theoretical construct or trait (e.g. intelligence, personality, foot posture).

CONTENT VALIDITY

Content validity refers to how well a test measures the behaviour for which it is intended, i.e. the test measures what it is supposed to measure.

CONTINUOUS VARIABLE

A continuous variable is one that can take on many values in a continuous order. Examples would be age, income, number of medication errors, score on a test.

CONTROL GROUP

A group of participants involved in a trial who receive either no intervention or the current best available, as is appropriate. This helps provide information on the additional benefit over nothing, or a new treatment over the current best treatment.

CORRELATION

The degree to which the scores on two variables co-relate, i.e. the extent to which a variation in the scores on the first variable results in a corresponding variation in the scores on the second variable.

CRITICAL APPRAISAL

A process of systematically and rigorously appraising published research to determine whether it is (a) internally valid, and therefore capable of providing useful information, and (b) externally valid, and therefore capable of providing information that can be applied to populations (groups of patients) outside the study.

CROSS–OVER TRIAL

In a cross-over trial each group receives the different treatments in turn. There may be a break between treatments so that the first drugs, or interventions, are cleared from the body before starting the next treatment.

DEPENDENT VARIABLE

The variable measured by the researcher and predicted to be influenced by the independent variable.

DIMENSION (of an issue, or clinical or theoretical problem)

A great majority of clinical and theoretical issues have multiple dimensions, i.e. different aspects to them. For example, if we are interested in the effectiveness of functional orthoses, there are various ways in which we can answer this question: we can evaluate technical success (influence on plantar pressure distribution, rearfoot motion or muscle activity), clinical success (pain reduction, improvements in function) or economic success (are orthoses cost-effective?). Each of these areas represents a dimension of the question.

DISCRETE VARIABLE

Variable with possible scores of discrete points on the scale. For example, number of children in a household – you can have 1, 2, 3 or 4 but not 3.45.

DISSEMINATION

A process that can involve a range of techniques by which research results and findings are communicated with interested individuals/professions/organizations. Example methods of dissemination include publications, conference presentations and press releases.

DISTRIBUTION

An arrangement of values of a variable showing their observed or theoretical frequency of occurrence. The most frequent term discussed is the so-called 'normal distribution' which is a theoretical frequency distribution for a set of data, usually represented by a bell-shaped curve symmetrical about the mean. Hence, the most frequent value is the mean and there are approximately equal numbers above and below the mean.

DOE

Acronym that stands for 'disease-oriented evidence'. Term coined by Slawson and Shaugnessy to describe the kind of article that is least relevant for physicians to know about, because it uses intermediate or disease-oriented outcomes. This kind of evidence should not change or guide practice because it is premature.

DOUBLE-BLIND TRIAL

see Blinding.

EPIDEMIOLOGY

The study of the incidence, distribution and determinants of disease, in an effort to understand cause. This is a key step in identifying opportunities for treatment and prevention.

EVIDENCE-BASED MEDICINE/EVIDENCE-BASED PRACTICE

A process devised to help clinicians practise optimally. A five-step process, it involves the formulation of a focused question, an efficient literature review to find useful information, critical appraisal of the evidence identified and subsequent modifications to practice, and audit of the outcome of any changes in practice.

EXTERNAL VALIDITY

Relates to the ability to apply findings from a particular research study to a wider population. If a study is externally valid, it means that the findings can be applied to a wider population.

FALSE NEGATIVE

In relation to diagnostic tests, a false negative refers to a situation where the test result states that a particular pathology is not present, when in fact it is.

FALSE POSITIVE

In relation to diagnostic tests, a false positive refers to a situation where the test result states that a particular pathology is present, when in fact it is not.

GENERALIZABILITY

Related to external validity – the ability to apply the findings of a research study to a wider population. Another way of stating this is to say that the results can be generalized to others.

GREY LITERATURE

Material that usually is available through specialized channels but may not enter normal channels or system of publications.

HETEROGENEITY (of a sample or group)

A sample is said to be heterogeneous when there is considerable variation in it. For example, a group which has children, adults and the elderly in it is more heterogeneous than a group of any one of these by themselves. Heterogeneity within a group equates with variation, which can be a weakness, as it can obscure an important relationship with any of the individual groups.

HOMOGENEITY (of a sample or group)

A sample is said to be homogeneous if it is similar, with minimal variation. For example, if a study was conducted on a group of children, it was conducted on a more homogeneous group than a study that involved participants of any age. Homogeneity is relative, however, as 'children' could be a group ranging from 2 to 16, or from 8 to 12.

HYPOTHESIS (descriptive and directional)

The hypothesis is a statement about the relationship between variables and this is what gets tested in any research study. Every experiment has two hypotheses: the null hypothesis states that there is no change or difference as a result of the independent variable, e.g. clinical practice does not result in a difference in clinical skills. The alternative hypothesis states that there is a change or difference, e.g. more clinical practice results in better clinical skills. When we perform statistics, we are always testing for the null and therefore results of any statistical procedures are always stated in regard to the null hypothesis.

INCIDENCE

The number of new cases of a disorder or disease occurring in a specified population in a specified time period. For example, we can measure the incidence of avian flu in South-East Asia in 2006.

INDEPENDENT VARIABLE

Any variable that you believe might influence your outcome measure (or dependent variable). This might be a variable that you control (e.g. a treatment) or a variable not under your control (e.g. an exposure). It might also represent a demographic factor such as age or gender.

INTERNAL VALIDITY

A study that is internally valid has employed sufficient methodological design features to allow it to provide valid information relating to the aim that was set.

LIKERT SCALE   A type of response format used in surveys developed by Rensis Likert. Likert items have responses on a continuum and response categories such as 'strongly agree', 'agree', 'disagree' and 'strongly disagree'.

LITERATURE REVIEW   A careful search of various information sources to find knowledge relating to a particular topic. Almost always involves an electronic, searchable database, but may also involve hand-searching journals which are not cited in a database. The aim is to identify information that will provide a balanced, objective perspective on the topic of interest.

MATCHING   In case-control studies this involves ensuring that the cases and controls are similar (i.e. matched) in important ways. For example, age, sex, occupation or recreational activities may be responsible for differences between two groups if they are not 'matched'.

MEAN   The mean is a measure of average (along with median and mode). The mean is the most common measure of mathematical average. To calculate the mean, add up all the terms and then divide by the number of terms.

MEASUREMENT ERRORS   These are errors which occur when taking measurements. There are two forms of measurement error: random error (e.g. mood of person) and systematic error (e.g. any factors that systematically affect measurement). Any investigator needs to reduce systematic error.

MeSH (Medical Subject Headings)   A highly structured thesaurus index.

META-ANALYSIS   This is a complex statistical technique which refers to the combination and analysis of multiple similar studies. Individual studies are collated and analysed with the purpose of integrating the findings.

MOOSE GUIDELINES   An acronym for a guideline relating to the evaluation of observational studies. MOOSE = **M**eta-analysis **O**f **O**bservational **S**tudies in **E**pidemiology.

MORBIDITY   Negative health effects, excepting death, are referred to as morbidity. For example, there is significant morbidity associated with hip fractures, i.e. detrimental health effects.

MORTALITY   Mortality refers to death. Just as there is significant morbidity associated with hip fractures, there is also significant mortality – some patients die as a result.

MULTI-DIMENSIONAL   Every issue, or clinical or theoretical problem, has multiple dimensions, i.e. 'aspects'. For example, the question: 'Are functional foot orthoses effective' has many dimensions. Are they technically effective (at improving plantar pressures, foot motion or muscular activity), are they clinically effective (at improving pain levels or activity levels) or economically effective (do they provide an efficient cost/benefit ratio). Technical, clinical and economic efficacy can be considered 'dimensions' to the issue of the effectiveness of orthoses.

NECESSARY CAUSE

A causal variable which *must* be present and acting in order for a disease to develop. A typical example relates to infectious disease where exposure to the human immunodeficiency virus must occur for AIDS to develop.

NICE

The National Institute for Health and Clinical Excellence is the independent organization responsible for providing national guidance on the promotion of good health and the prevention and treatment of ill health.

OBSERVATIONAL STUDIES

Studies which involve observing, or measuring, characteristics in a population. This type of study serves to provide information on the natural history of a disease. No intervention is undertaken.

ORDINAL VARIABLES

Similar to a categorical variable although there is one significant difference: with ordinal variables there is a clear ordering of the variables. For example, suppose you have a variable, educational experience: no qualifications, GCSEs, A levels, degrees, postgraduate degrees. We can order these variables, but we cannot say that the interval between them is the same (if we could, then the variable would be an interval variable).

PILOT STUDY

The initial, preliminary study examining a new method or treatment. A brief, smaller study that can help you iron out any problems with the study before you conduct the main study.

PLACEBO (group)

A dummy treatment intervention (e.g. a pill) which is physiologically inactive. Permits analysis of 'mind over matter' – the possibility that it is simply interest in the patient that is stimulating. A placebo group receives the placebo intervention.

POEM

Acronym that stands for 'patient-oriented evidence that matters'. Term coined by Slawson and Shaugnessy to describe the kind of article that is most relevant for physicians to know about, because it uses patient-oriented outcomes, deals with a problem that we see in our practice, and has the potential to change the way we practice.

POWER (of a study)

In planning a new study, researchers use power analysis to increase their odds of finding the true result or effect that is present. In medicine, for example, power analyses provide critical information when planning large-scale clinical trials, especially when the incidence rate of a disease or drug side effect is small.

PREVALENCE

The number of cases of a disorder or disease present in a specific population at a specific point in time. As regards the relationship between prevalence and incidence (the number of cases occurring over a specific time period in a specific population), chronic diseases may have a low incidence but a high prevalence (due to fatality being rare), whilst acute, life-threatening illnesses may have a high incidence but a low prevalence (due to a high mortality rate).

PROBABILITY	At its most simple, probability is the likelihood that something will happen. For example, a probability of less than 0.05 indicates that the probability of something occurring by chance alone is less than 5 in 100, or 5%. The abbreviation for probability is p. Obviously, the lower the p value, the less likely the event has happened by chance and is a real change.
PROTOCOL	A step-by-step guide to the method used in a study. A clear, detailed protocol serves as a user guide that permits a study to be repeated.
QUALITATIVE RESEARCH	Research that involves the investigation of attitudes, beliefs or experiences. In a study evaluating the effectiveness of orthoses, qualitative information would relate to ease of use, the hassle associated with using orthoses and the effect that such problems had on patients.
QUANTITATIVE RESEARCH	Research that involves 'hard' measurement, such as blood pressure, shoe size, weight or height. Such measurements tend to be more repeatable and more rapidly obtained than qualitative information.
RANDOMIZATION	A process whereby individuals eligible for inclusion within an interventional trial are allocated to receive either of the treatment options. Equates with a process similar to the throw of a dice and should be totally objective. The object is to ensure that any unknown factors are equally distributed between treatment groups in an effort to reduce bias.
RANDOMIZED CONTROLLED TRIAL (RCT)	A research design that represents the gold standard for investigating the effect of a treatment. Eligible participants are randomly allocated to receive simply treatment 'A' or treatment 'B' and ideally neither the patient nor the researcher knows who is receiving what. This means that the placebo effect and any influence originating from the researcher can be reduced.
RELIABILITY	When taking measurements we need to be sure that in the absence of a true change in the variable being measured, we will obtain the same value each time we take the measurement. High reliability means that the results being obtained with successive measurements are very close. Poor reliability occurs when there is high variation between successive measurements.
REPEATABILITY	A term that is often used when referring to reliability. Carries the same meaning.
RESEARCH	Defined by the Department of Health as: 'Rigorous and systematic enquiry conducted on a scale and using methods commensurate with the issues investigated and designed to lead to generalizable contributions to knowledge.'
RESEARCH GOVERNANCE	Refers to a governance of research that utilizes the principles of high-quality ethical research in health and social care. It is the key to ensuring research is conducted legally to high methodological and ethical standards.

RESEARCH GOVERNANCE PROCESSES

Validity, reliability, generalizability, appropriateness and bias.

SAMPLE SIZE

The sample size is very simply the size of the sample. If there is only one sample, the letter 'N' is used to designate the sample size; if samples are taken from each of 'a' populations, then the letter 'n' is used to designate the size of the sample from each population.

SAMPLE SIZE CALCULATION

Research studies (surveys, experiments, observational studies, etc.) are always better when they are carefully planned and one aspect of careful planning is to obtain an adequate sample size. The sample size must be 'big enough' that an effect of such magnitude as to be of scientific significance will also be statistically significant. It is just as important, however, that the study not be 'too big', where an effect of little scientific importance is nevertheless statistically detectable. There are a number of mathematical methods and formulae that can be used to calculate the sample size.

SENSITIVITY

(1) Of a diagnostic test: refers to the proportion of people with disease who have a positive test result. If sensitivity is high, a negative result rules the diagnosis out. (2) Of a literature search: the proportion of all relevant studies in the database retrieved by a literature search.

SINGLE–BLIND TRIAL

see Blinding.

SPECIFICITY

(1) Of a diagnostic test: refers to the proportion of people without disease who have a negative test result. If specificity is high, a positive result rules the diagnosis in. (2) Of a literature search: the proportion of all studies retrieved by a literature search that are relevant.

STANDARD DEVIATION

The standard deviation is a statistic that tells you how tightly all the values are clustered around the mean in a set of data. Hence, a small standard deviation suggests that most values are close to the mean, whereas a large standard deviation suggests that the values range widely from the mean.

STATISTICAL SIGNIFICANCE

A finding is described as statistically significant when it can be demonstrated that the probability of obtaining such a difference only by chance is relatively low. It is customary to describe one's finding as statistically significant when the obtained result is among those that (theoretically) would occur no more than 5 times out of 100 by chance (i.e. $p < 0.05$).

STROBE GUIDELINES

Guidelines concerning the evaluation of observational studies. STROBE = **S**trengthening **T**he **R**eporting of **Ob**servational Studies in **E**pidemiology. Comprises a series of questions through which the quality of an observational study can be evaluated.

SUFFICIENT CAUSE

A causal factor which, by itself, is capable of inducing a disease or disorder. In heart disease, there are many risk factors that can act alone or together. However, any individual factor capable of inducing the disease by itself can be termed a 'sufficient' cause.

SYSTEMATIC REVIEW

Exactly what it states: a literature review that adopts a standardized approach to literature searching in an attempt to be as rigorous as possible (although it does not necessarily claim to be comprehensive). All research studies identified are then appraised according to standardized criteria to permit objective analysis of quality.

TYPE I ERROR

One of the two errors it is possible to make after conducting a research study. All research studies aim to gather information relating to a hypothesis. If we reject a null hypotheses on the basis of the data gathered when it is actually true, then this is termed a type I error. A simple example would be when an ultrasound scan says that a patient has a neuroma when in fact they do not.

TYPE II ERROR

The second error it is possible to make after conducting a research study. All research studies aim to gather information relating to a hypothesis. If we accept the null hypothesis on the basis of the data gathered when it is actually true, then this is termed a type II error. A simple example would be a situation where we fail to identify a difference when there actually is one.

VALIDITY

Broadly speaking refers to 'truth'. If a blood pressure monitor measures 140/70, and this is actually the subject's blood pressure, then the monitor is valid. This is a vital concept: we must use valid measurement techniques as these ensure the quality of the information on which to base practice.

WILDCARDS

In literature, allow for searches to look for several variations of the same word by substituting letters in the middle of the word with a single character.

Appendix 1

Electronic resources

The internet provides many resources of value to healthcare professionals. Topics covered include evidence-based practice, clinical governance, research methods and statistics. This guide is not intended to be comprehensive; rather, it is a focused guide to some of the best resources available. What follows is a link to what we consider to be essential websites that are 'treasure troves' of information. We suggest that you take a few hours to go through these sites one by one, considering what each offers, and bookmark those that particularly appeal. These are authoritative, respected websites. If you are a student, don't drive your tutors to despair by passing these over in favour of obscure sites when researching assignments!

Please note that at the time of publication the web addresses were all current. However, given the nature of the internet it is highly likely that some of these may change or be removed. If the address does not seem to work a search using the website name should identify it if it is still available.

Website	Address	Description
ADEPT	www.shef.ac.uk/scharr/ir/adept	An online tutorial covering applied diagnosis, aetiology, therapy and prognosis. Particularly useful is a guide to ensuring that literature searches only look for evidence-based research
Bandolier	www.jr2.ox.ac.uk/bandolier	A superb site that aims to simplify the process of evidence-based practice. Provides a host of features including superb 'What is...' guides which cover a range of topics related to EBP
Centre for Evidence-Based Medicine (Oxford)	www.cebm.net	Website of one of the more prominent EBP centres in the world
Centre for Evidence-Based Medicine (Toronto)	www.cebm.utoronto.ca	As above – the Oxford and Toronto centres are leading lights in the world of EBM

Note that there are many other regional 'centres for evidence-based practice'

(Continued)

Website	Address	Description
Centre for Reviews and Dissemination, York University	www.york.ac.uk/inst/crd	York University has a large team working on EBP projects and systematic reviews. The website provides access to searchable databases of pre-appraised evidence such as DARE: Database of Reviews of Effectiveness. Clinical access to this database offers a useful source of evidence for rapidly informing clinical decision-making
Clinical Evidence	www.clinicalevidence.com/ceweb/index.jsp	A monthly updated directory of evidence on the effects of common clinical interventions
Clinical governance in primary care	www.eldis.org/static/DOC11531.htm	Provides information about the initiative aimed at improving the quality of care and accountability in the NHS
Clinical Governance Bulletin	www.rsmpress.co.uk/cgb.htm	Free, bimonthly, publication on best practice in clinical governance. Adobe Acrobat required
Clinical Governance – Resource pack	www.wisdomnet.co.uk/clingov.asp	Useful resource pack with links to various useful resources
Clinical Effectiveness (NHS Executive)	www.wisdomnet.co.uk/clingov.asp	NHS Executive page with links to booklet and resource pack on clinical effectiveness
Cochrane Collaboration	www.cochrane.org/index.htm	Home site of the international effort to produce, maintain and disseminate systematic reviews of evidence about the prevention and treatment or control of health problems
Critical Appraisal Skills Programme	www.phru.nhs.uk/casp/casp.htm	Homepage of an excellent, and influential, resource for critical appraisal. Recommended by Oxford Centre for Evidence-Based Medicine
Evidence-based Healthcare and Public Health (journal)	www.harcourt-international.com/journals/ebhc	Table of contents and abstracts concerning a range of issues in EBP
Evidence-based Medicine and Audit Portal	www.openclinical.org/ebm.html	Provides links to sites related to EBP, healthcare informatics and audit
Evidence-based medicine (GP Notebook)	www.gpnotebook.co.uk/simplepage.cfm?ID=-1596981199	Evidence-based information on a range of medical conditions, from the GP Notebook service
Health Evidence Bulletins (Wales)	hebw.cf.ac.uk	Regular update on best current evidence across a broad range of evidence types and subject areas from mental health to health environments
National Institute for Health and Clinical Excellence	www.nice.org.uk	Website of the (in)famous organization charged with providing the NHS in England and Wales with authoritative, robust and reliable guidance on current 'best practice'
National Library for Health	www.library.nhs.uk	Formerly the National electronic Library for Health, this is the NHS 'storefront' for information resources for its staff. A one-stop gateway to many of the resources listed here, from Bandolier to the Cochrane Library and Clinical Governance. Also provides 'professional portals' – links to resources aimed at specific AHPs

(Continued)

Website	Address	Description
Scottish Intercollegiate Guidelines Network (SIGN)	www.sign.ac.uk	SIGN develops and publishes evidence-based clinical practice guidelines for use by the health service in Scotland

In addition to these resources, various critical appraisal/research methodology websites exist. These provide a very useful and focused insight to the optimum research designs in various areas. They are:

- *ASSERT*: A Standard for the Scientific and Ethical Review of Trials – www.assert-statement.org
- *The CONSORT Statement*: Consolidated Standards for Reporting Trials – www.consort-statement.org
- *MOOSE*: Meta-Analysis of Observational Studies in Epidemiology – www.consort-statement.org/Initiatives/MOOSE/moose.pdf
- *STARD Initiative*: Towards complete and accurate reporting of studies of diagnostic accuracy – www.consort-statement.org/stardstatement.htm
- *STROBE*: Strengthening the Reporting of Observational Studies in Epidemiology – www.strobe-statement.org

Index